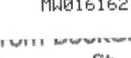
The 3 Keys to Conception

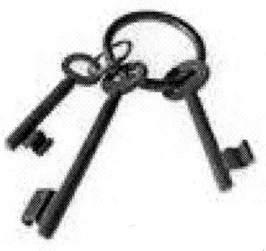

Lynsi Eastburn

COPYRIGHT

©2013 Lynsi Eastburn

For information contact Eastburn Hypnotherapy Center
7905 N. Zenobia St.
Westminster, CO 80030
303-424-2331
office@hypnodenver.com ~ www.hypnodenver.com

Order this book online at www.tatteredcover.com
or at major online book retailers.

Printed in the United States of America.

ISBN: 978-1-938859-20-5

D. James Publishing
Tattered Cover Press

www.hypnofertility.com ~ www.spiritbabywhisperer.com

"One thing that comes out of myth is that at the bottom of the abyss comes the voice of salvation. The black moment is the moment when the real message of transformation is going to come. At the darkest moment comes the light."

—Joseph Campbell

Dedication

This book is dedicated to the mothers who have influenced me in loving ways, in positive ways. They have helped weave the intricate web that is my destiny–some for a moment, some for a lifetime–and I couldn't have done it without them.

With top billing to my "actual" mother:

Nancy Carter
Otti Gloger
Anna Marie Fidel-Rice
WhiteOak
Martie O'Brien
Brenda Lynne Ross
Sue Thomas
Albertine Brûlé
Marilyn Leidecker

I must also include here my sister, Sharron Carter Vasilakos– we learned those early ropes together . . . she, and only she.

I hereby recognize and appreciate those who have been instrumental in the creation of this work:

My husband & soul mate, Drake Eastburn
& our beloved dogs Scout & Boo Radley

My Sons & Daughters (in one way or another)

Kelly Brûlé & Zoe Swanson
Dylan Brûlé & Kaitlin Henderson
Coady Brûlé, Kylie Fauth & New Baby Son
Candace Brûlé & Davan Ramkissoon

Editors & Consultants

Melanie, Steve, Molly & Ryan Brady (Foreword)
Drake Eastburn ~ Jack Fields
Molly Jenkins ~ Martie O'Brien

Cover Design

Martie O'Brien

Support & Inspiration (to name only a few)

Luke, Chris & George Vasilakos; Joe Gloger;
Mark & Suzy Eastburn; Teri Buller;
The Leideckers: Art, Reene & Christian; Tracy Johnston;
Dr. Mark Bush & staff–Conceptions Repro.
Dr. Dwight Damon et al–National Guild of Hypnotists
My students, clients and spirit babies–past, present & future

And Special Acknowledgement to

Rob & Karen Gloger

A Few Words from the Author

You've heard of the term "chick flick." I kinda like to think of this as a "chick book." Though men are most certainly part of the fertility process, there is something here that is somehow primal, something to be shared by the divine goddesses that live within each one of us–that ARE each one of us. This is a chance to pull on some comfy pajamas, scatter some fluffy pillows and snuggly blankets across the floor, and settle in for a heart to heart, girl to girl, woman to woman, goddess to goddess play date of sorts. An intimate exchange that reaps much needed nurturing and support for all involved.

Mothers, daughters, grandmothers . . . sisters, cousins, aunts . . . Powerful women encircling each other–maybe one or two, maybe hundreds or more gathered together in this haven we are creating . . . now. The wondrous feminine element: past, present, future; physical world or spirit. All are welcome. For a little while, at least, all bonds are broken, we are fluid and free. The ambiance: candles perhaps. Soothing music. Blessed rose oil–the scent of the Divine Mother. In honor of the ultimate feminine: body, mind, and spirit; connected.

Thank you for being here . . .

In Love, Light & Peace,

–Lynsi Eastburn

December 30, 2012

ix

SPONSORS

Heartfelt thanks goes out to the following individuals whose dedication to—and support of—this essential healing work helps to sustain the ever evolving process . . .

In gratitude, love, and peace we present:

Shelley Torgove, Clinical Herbalist

Artemisia & Rue
Telephone: 303-484-8982
www.artemesiaandrue.com
shelley@artemesiaandrue.com

Shelley is a practicing Clinical Herbalist, trained Fertility Awareness Instructor and Certified Massage Therapist. She is a nationally recognized botanical medicine practitioner and teacher with over 20 years of experience, specializing in herbal medicine for women, fertility issues and menstrual cycle problems.

Shelley is the owner of Artemisia & Rue, an herbal pharmacy and retail store focusing on therapeutic uses of herbal medicines, essential oils, pure aromatic perfumes, tincture preparations, custom formulations and community herb classes. Shelley and her husband Daniel Pool-Pech offer professional level training programs and apprenticeships in Western herbal medicine and traditional Maya healing practices- both in Colorado and in Tulum, Mexico.

Shelley was one of the first students trained in Maya Abdominal Massage by Dr. Rosita Arvigo, Hortence Robinson and Beatrice Waight in Belize. Each year she leads students to Mexico to study traditional healing practices. She graduated from the Southwest School of Botanical Medicine in 1993 where she studied under Michael Moore and Donna Chesner. Shelley is eternally grateful to many other mentors including: Aviva Gold for her Painting from The Source work; Ann Drucker and her earth-centered herbalism and shamanism teachings; Adam Seller and Cascade Anderson-Geller for sharing their herbal wisdom and love of 'materia medica'; most recently Lynsi Eastburn for her powerful HypnoFertility® training and Estela Roman and Daniel Pool-Pech for their ongoing teachings of traditional medicine—both Aztec and Maya.

Shelley loves traveling world, and enjoys conversing in Spanish daily. Her other interests include gathering plants in wild places and spending time playing with her daughter.

The Rev. Dr. C. Scot Giles, D.Min., LLC

1211 Pershing Avenue
Wheaton, Illinois 60189
Telephone: 630-668-1141
ScotGiles@comcast.net
www.CSGiles.org

The Rev. Dr. C. Scot Giles is a Board Certified Chaplain and the Board Certified Diplomate of the National Guild of Hypnotists. His practice is a specialty practice in medical hypnotism that is known around the world. He works in conjunction with several Chicago area hospitals and wellness centers, including the University of Chicago Medical Center. He works with clients over Skype from around the nation.

Akiko Yokoyama, MD, PhD, CH

Yokoyama Clinic
Miyazaki, Japan
http://yokoyama-clinic.net
info@yokoyama-clinic.net

Akiko Yokoyama is a medical doctor, PHD, and a NGH certified hypnotherapist. She has had special training in parts therapy, age regression hypnotherapy, past life therapy, and Lynsi's HypnoFertility® program. In her own clinic, she runs a general private hypnotherapy practice with an emphasis on HypnoFertility®. Akiko also works as a "Kampo" medicine doctor in an IVF clinic. "Kampo" is a Japanese traditional herbal medicine. She wants to support women, especially women with infertility, from many aspects including hypnotherapy, Kampo herbal medicine, and yoga. Akiko is the first medical doctor who practices HypnoFertility® in Japan.

Ingrid Zirnis Johnson

Z Hypnotherapy
Boulder, CO
www.ZHypnotherapy.com
Telephone: 303-776-8100
Member, Boulder Chamber of Commerce
Certified Hypnotherapist, Gestalt-Based Hypnotherapist & HypnoFertility® Consultant, MIR Method Practitioner

HypnoFertility® practitioner and hypnotherapist, Ingrid combines an extensive background in coaching and natural health. Drawing on international certification from the Pacific Institute of Aromatherapy, certification from Five Elements Center for Homeopathy, certification from the Foundation for Shamanic Studies (and a sustaining member), as well as Yuen Energetics, Psych-K, EFT, and the MIR Method, gives Ingrid a broad base for achieving optimum results for her clients.

As a certified hypnotherapist and member of the National Guild of Hypnotists, Ingrid incorporates advanced training in Gestalt-Based Hypnotherapy with her 'listening to what's underneath the words' expertise. Sessions available in beautiful Boulder, CO setting, as well as long distance options.

Anne L. Walters, CNM, MSN

All About Women's Health Care P.C.
Englewood & Littleton, CO
Telephone: 303-781-5299

Anne Walters has been in practice since 1993 and is devoted to providing great healthcare to women of all ages. Besides standard midwifery care, she uses essential oil therapy, hypnosis, Mayan abdominal massage, magnetics and Far infrared therapy as needed.

Jenet Kirby

Deep Thoughts Hypnotherapy
Melbourne, Australia
Telephone: Australia 03 9530 4690
International: +61 3 9530 4690
Mobile: Australia 0400 538 621
International: +61400 538 621
www.deepthoughtshypnotherapy.com.au
E-mail: jenet@deepthoughtshypnotherapy.com.au

Jenet Kirby is a Clinical Hypnotherapist specializing in Women's Health and Wellbeing. Since starting as a nurse in 1975, she has trained in Australia and overseas as a Certified HypnoFertility® Therapist. As well, Jenet trained as a HypnoBirthing® Childbirth Educator and is certified in Medical Hypnotherapy.

Having given birth herself, Jenet has a special interest in this wonderful experience and now is thrilled to be a grandmother. In her private practice, Jenet's areas of expertise include smoking cessation, stress management, pain control, phobia reduction, weight loss and diabetes management. There are many other areas too numerous to list here.

Trained in the Sheila Granger—Virtual Gastric Band Procedure for reducing weight, Jenet knows that it may assist with improving health issues including increasing fertility. Self-hypnosis workshops conducted by Jenet, in Melbourne and the rural areas, enable both men and women to enjoy and enrich their lives.

Jenet is accredited as a clinical member of the Australian Hypnotherapists' Association (AHA) as well as a professional clinical member of the Australian Association of Clinical Hypnotherapy & Psychotherapy, Inc. (AACHP). She is also a full member of the National Guild of Hypnotists.

Angelika Baum, CHt, DAc

5865 Dalebrook Cres., Unit 25B
Mississauga, Ontario
L5M 5X1
Telephone: 905-286-9466
greendoorrelaxation@yahoo.ca
www.greendoorrelaxation.net

Angelika is a Certified Hypnotist, Acupuncturist, and Life Coach focusing on belief changes. Having had to personally overcome "unexplained infertility," Angelika is very passionate about helping other women in the same situation. She holds certifications in a range of different areas of hypnosis but specializes in conception, pregnancy, and birth.

Angelika is a member of the National Guild of Hypnotists. She has had a full-time hypnosis practice since 2004, and added Psych-K® to her repertoire in 2006. She trained with Lynsi Eastburn in 2009 and has since assisted many couples in overcoming their fertility issues. Her CDs "Stress-free Conception" and "Hypnosis for Fertility" are available through her website.

Jenn Price-Jones

Calgary, Alberta, Canada
www.CalgaryHypnoFertility.com
www.CalgaryHealingHypnosis.com
Telephone: 403-816-7155

Jenn Price-Jones is a Certified Hypnotherapist with the National Guild of Hypnotists (since 2000). She has been certified with Lynsi Eastburn as a Certified HypnoFertility® Therapist. A HypnoBirthing® practitioner since 2001, Jenn is also trained as a Doula, in EFT, as a Life Coach, and in Somatic Healing with David Quigley, as well as several other modalities. Her goal is helping people to improve their lives, helping women become pregnant and/or to have joyous, natural, gentle births.

Tanya Zappia

Northglenn, Colorado
Telephone: 616-443-8566
yasistatanya@yahoo.com

Tanya is a practicing Life Coach and student of *A Course in Miracles*. Most of her life coaching has been with teens and young adults, guiding them to use responsibility, honesty and integrity when making choices in their lives. Tanya's life coaching experiences with adults have helped her to grow as much as those she's worked with, discovering and realizing more potential and less resistance. Tanya enjoys sharing lessons and experiences pertaining to the *Course* with fellow students, as well as living as an example of what the *Course* teaches.

TABLE OF CONTENTS

What I faced was daunting: a seven-year holding pattern with the diagnosis of unexplained infertility; seven unsuccessful IUIs; two failed IVFs—the last resulting in a miscarriage days after a positive pregnancy test. Reminders were everywhere and I'd break into tears at the sight of a pregnant belly, baby or family . . . My doctor said, "You're putting too much faith in science." I knew it was not God's plan—or mine—for me to be childless, so I put my faith there too, but I was impatient with His seven-year lesson to teach me patience. My husband, Steve, and I were devastated but we were also committed, committed to focusing on us and committed to building our family. Our savings drained, our credit cards maxed, he took a weekend job and secured private consulting gigs in addition to our full-time work. Time was ticking. We decided after rebuilding some of our savings, we'd adopt. It was still daunting but we weren't done.

We set February 1, 2011 as our start date. In January, we posted on Facebook and adoption websites of our desire to adopt a newborn—we had always thought that we'd have a boy and a girl named Molly and Ryan—and we called an agency to review the process and fees. Then, on February 1st, as I sat down to complete background checks, criminal clearances, and fingerprint forms for the FBI, my phone rang. A nurse rattled off the biographical details of a man and a woman—excuse me, what is this? My mind reeled: it was the fertility clinic where we had sought a second opinion a year before.

I remembered answering in the affirmative when the doctor asked if we were open to frozen embryo adoption. On February 1st, our names had reached the top of their recipient waitlist. The striking thing was we weren't even completely aware that our names had been placed on the list, as there was nothing to sign. I stood, intuitively aware of the remarkable coincidence that two sibling embryos would come to us on this date, awed too by the sunbeams shining through my skylight, and the full feeling of a miracle enveloping me. I called Steve.

This was it. A miracle had happened. Our babies answered our advertisement.

Would my body accept these beautiful blastocysts and get pregnant on our tenth try at assisted reproduction? Lynsi's first book, *It's Conceivable!*, was the first that I had heard about hypnotherapy, let alone the idea of preparing the mind as well as the body for pregnancy. Intrigued, I looked for a local Board Certified Hypnotherapist. But I kept returning to her biography, the expert who had literally written the book on the subject. She was the best. And I needed the best for the sake of these two precious babies waiting to be born.

I wanted a similar experience to those Lynsi had chronicled—purging obstacles and meeting my internal assistant. I imagined myself resting in the beanbag that I had read about in her office. I wanted to tell her everything, succinctly, to come clean, get it all off my chest, confide, confess, and cry. She listened over the phone as I blurted out my story through snotty sobs. "Our session is your time to fill-up the metaphorical sink," she said. "When we hang up, you will pull the sink stopper and all the disappointment and doubt and negative thinking will go down the drainpipe." The actual hypnosis—a personalized audio file sent via email—weaved elements of our conversation into a new positive focus on the future, healing, and preparing for pregnancy.

At first, I was dubious, having only seen hypnosis as stage acts in the movies. I worried that I was too alert, trying too hard. Then I focused on Lynsi's soothing voice and followed her words to let every muscle go limp, release all thoughts, and take nice deep breaths. When I released my anxieties and expectations, I saw—and let me preface before I describe my vision that I was not an angel fanatic—gigantic, beautiful rough feathery angelic wings, huge, pink with deep brown patterns, swooping in close to me and holding two babies; I could see their pudgy legs and booties in her hands. Hands that were extended, palms up, the babies sitting in them, and as the feathers got closer and closer to me, the extended hands, almost in prayer position, pointed toward my uterus and gave the babies to me. I felt elated. I shared my vision with Lynsi after my session. "You are an enlightened witness, this is fantastic! The universe is generous. Accept that you can have what you want." That night, as per Lynsi's script, I had a deep, luxurious sleep, a rejuvenating sleep, like never before.

In her new book, Lynsi describes the *3 Keys to Conception*. Through shared turning points, we learn more about what drew Lynsi into this field, her remarkable connection to "spirit babies," that these babies are her actual clients uniquely bringing their chosen parents to her. The book illustrates the importance of meditation, trusting in the process, and listening to the universe for the necessary balance of mind-body-spirit, prerequisites for women who have struggled with infertility to achieve healthy pregnancy.

My own pregnancy was protected by my "personal assistant" like the ones Lynsi had written about in *It's Conceivable!* I was prepared for a tiny nurse, hopefully not a spider, maybe an elephant . . . when who should present herself but Tinker Bell. I was embarrassed to admit this to Lynsi, feeling as though my imagination had taken an easy out, especially when I began noticing all the commercial merchandise with Tinker Bell's image. But Lynsi reassured me, "your subconscious mind gets it, the silly factor doesn't matter, a fairy, a cartoon—it is whatever nourishes the mind, and the mind is impacted by images. It is now a foregone conclusion that your mind is shifting from infertility to fertility; don't limit your mind, don't try to figure out all the details, your subconscious mind already sees the end result."

I made peace with Tink; after all, she wore a green dress—the color of fertility—and we had similar features so I came to think of her as a mini-me in a sense, though she definitely had her own identity and role to play that became very real to me. After I asked Tink to supervise my uterine polyp removal surgery, I woke in recovery Room #4 and saw Tink floating in my lap and giving me the thumbs up. I laughed, still feeling the effects of the general anesthesia, at what would have been an odd hallucination before my hypnotherapy.

Tink was there at my embryo transfer, accepting both blastocysts and sewing them into my nutritious and welcoming uterine lining, where they would "bloom and grow" in their amniotic sacs, the thread coming out like stitches when ready, and Tink flying around the small spaces where I couldn't see to inspect that everything was secure. She was also there when I was hospitalized with bleeding from a potential placenta previa—and Lynsi guided me on how to shut the bleeding off via an internal faucet. "The hypnosis recordings are in your psyche, that is your new default," Lynsi said. "When a negative thought seeps in, you know it is just a thought and recognize it for what it is and let it go. You have powerful tools this time that you didn't have last time."

Molly and Ryan were indeed born, early yet healthy, on January 12, 2012. I am honored and forever changed by my hypnotherapy experience with Lynsi. I readily agreed to write this foreword because I am convinced that Molly and Ryan are here with us today thanks in large part to Lynsi and her work. She offers deep insight, a generous heart and a kind soul—and the spirit babies know it!

Best of luck in your HypnoFertility® journey,

Melanie Brady

Meditate

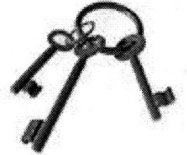

Chapter 1

IT'S CONCEIVABLE

"An idea, like a ghost . . . must be spoken to a little before it will explain itself."

—*Charles Dickens*

Approximately a dozen years or so ago, in my general hypnotherapy practice, I found myself consulting more and more frequently with women dealing with the devastating diagnosis of infertility. It started with a woman seeking assistance with a needle phobia that was preventing her from undergoing yet another in vitro fertilization cycle. Hypnosis is well recognized for its effectiveness with phobias such as this. And though it has also been utilized in childbirth for decades hypnotherapy for fertility was virtually unprecedented when I began working with it with increasing regularity in my private practice. Initially, clients not only released needle phobias or other anxiety related ailments, they also reported "night and day" responses to IVF cycles, an ability to "forget about it [their fertility issues] for a little while," as well as a sense of "getting their lives back."

I have always been one to pay attention to whatever comes my way. I believe that when something's time has come it virtually floods the collective unconscious and certain individuals can see it if they choose to. Before long I'd logged literally thousands of clinic hours utilizing hypnosis for fertility and developing my own program—which I dubbed HypnoFertility®—and which I began teaching to therapists and hypnotherapists worldwide in 2003. In 2005 I began writing my book, *It's Conceivable! Hypnosis for Fertility*, which I released in 2006.

It's Conceivable! was written for the public—it chronicles some of my client case studies and details many of the ways hypnosis can help with fertility issues. I wrote it so people would know that help is available and that hypnosis is a highly effective modality for those struggling with infertility. *It's Conceivable!* immediately sold thousands of copies worldwide and before I knew it I was not only seeing clients locally, but was being asked to please work with clients via telephone and, eventually, Skype.

Though I have trained several hundred therapists in my methods, this is a very small number in the scope of the entire world population. Not all of them are practicing, and some have styles so far from mine that clients don't feel they are experiencing the process as described in my books, lectures, or even by my office assistants when they call or e-mail for a referral. In these cases if we can't find a suitable HypnoFertility® (HF) practitioner, I am able to work with people myself by phone or Skype—provided I have an opening.

The evolution of my life purpose is exactly what it is, regardless of what others may or may not be doing. As I said before, once something reaches its time, it becomes apparent in the collective and may well be "created" many times over. There are certain people who resonate with me—clients and students—and my focus is with them. I have a unique interpretation and expression of the process; to me, it's a soul connection and not at all about the ego.

I did not set out to become some kind of infertility guru. I have been drawn to the healing arts since I was a small child and psychology, Reiki, meditation, and hypnotherapy are just some of the stepping stones along my path. I struggled with releasing *It's Conceivable!* because I knew it would skyrocket my career in the fertility direction and I wasn't quite sure that was right for me. I had to do a lot of soul searching and one day I underwent a *Life Purpose* hypnosis regression session to see if I was, indeed, on the right track with my fertility work. In a nutshell I learned through this powerful hypnotic process that I did need to publish *It's Conceivable!* without hesitation, without a doubt.

I will briefly recap the experience here as it is a precursor to the eventual inception of this book. I was hypnotized by a therapist in my office and guided to the place I call *The Between.* The Between is the place between lives—where we decide what it is we are going to accomplish during a given lifetime, where we contract out for our assignment (for more on this see *Sacred Contracts* by Caroline Myss or *Inspiration* by Wayne Dyer). There I found myself in an old fashioned library. There were many, many books but the main one that caught my attention was *It's Conceivable!* right there on the shelf in front of me.

One of my clients' babies was there and he showed me how a spirit baby was placed inside another of my clients. (The client I saw in this vision had been in the process of IVF at the time of my regression and shortly thereafter we received the confirmation call that she was pregnant.) Suddenly, the room was filled with babies, spirit babies, and they were telling me that they needed my help, that "the alignment was off" and they "needed help to connect with their parents in the physical world." I was astounded. I knew it was true on some level yet I was absolutely astounded.

After the regression I decided I would go ahead and publish the book. I debated including my regression experience—the left-brained, so-called rational part of me said, "No way, they'll think you're nuts!" Regardless, I decided to include the experience—after all it is the truth, and it was the catalyst in my embracing the next phase of my own journey. In the seven years since *It's Conceivable!* was published I have picked up the nickname of *Spirit Baby Whisperer* from some of my clients and students. It is actually an accurate depiction of my parent/baby connections (the term whisperer is applied to someone who has an uncanny ability to communicate with another sentient being: babies, horses, dogs, spirit babies, even ghosts—as in *Ghost Whisperer*, etc.) so I have elected to use the term in tandem with HypnoFertility®, as well as to further illustrate and expand upon my life's work.

Chapter 2

SPIRIT BABY WHISPERER

"Technology is not going to save us. Our computers, our tools,
our machines are not enough.
We have to rely on our intuition, our true being."

—*Joseph Campbell*

One day in November of 2009 I was sitting in session with one of my clients when a little round ball of light floated past my field of vision. I squinted, rubbed my eyes, and vaguely wondered if I were perhaps getting a migraine (though I didn't have any pain or other symptoms, I figured this had to be one of those auras associated with migraine headaches). A few days later it happened again, and in recalling the first incident I realized that it had not been a precursor to a migraine. Soon I was seeing little orbs of light on a regular basis, but, interestingly, only in my office and only during client sessions. It dawned on me that I was, in fact, seeing spirit babies, but, not considering myself a psychic, I decided I'd best keep the knowledge to myself. Around the same time I started getting stronger impressions of my clients' babies, and I began to make more frequent notes on their files: "girl" or "she" or "he" or "they" . . . I was now clearly sensing babies more obviously than ever, and before they'd even been conceived.

This was not unusual to me in that I had noticed early on in my fertility work that when clients had a sense of their babies they were usually right. Regardless of what any doctor said, I had always put more stock in my clients' impressions than in their doctors' diagnoses. Time and time again my clients' intuitions had proven right, while prognoses of zero percent chance of conception and other such bleak stances had proven wrong before my very eyes. I documented this in my earlier book, *It's Conceivable!*, and, truthfully, it is the reason I have pursued this work to the extent that I have. I'd always believed in them, I'd always stood up for them; why wouldn't I begin to see the energetic imprints of the darling little beings so loved and cherished by their mothers and fathers—my clients?

Not long after I'd released *It's Conceivable!* a colleague sent me an excerpt from a book called *Spirit Babies*. Apparently, as I was coming to terms with my role in the planet's fertility challenge, a man named Walter Makichen was walking a somewhat similar path that had inadvertently led him to communication with what he also referred to as *spirit babies*. A client of mine from LA sent me Walter's book as a gift not long after I'd received the initial excerpt, and through his writings I received powerful validation of my own vision during the writing of *It's Conceivable!* The spirit babies were giving Walter some of the same messages they had given me. I had never heard of Walter Makichen until well after my book was published—yet we could have been writing of shared experiences.

As Walter's book gained in popularity I encountered more and more women who had also had telephone sessions with him. Our work was different—Walter worked more as a psychic reader who gave people messages from their children-to-be, though he also provided meditations and/or chants for them to help with (what I call) alignment issues. I work with the art and science of hypnotism to help clients access the necessary mind/body/spirit balance that helps them become parents. I always integrated Walter's information into my client's sessions and found this to be yet one more piece of the puzzle they were struggling to solve. If they'd had a phone session with Walter it made sense to work with the information he'd given them, and my work genuinely complemented his.

I noticed that my impressions were typically in complete harmony with what Walter had told my clients (in cases where they'd spoken with him) and that often both mine and Walter's impressions did not match up with medical prognoses. This is not to say that the work I do is anti-medical—it's not. In fact, probably half the work I do is in conjunction with medical treatments. In fact, I have a symbiotic affiliation with what I believe is the top patient-centered clinic in the United States—if not the world: *Conceptions Reproductive Associates of Colorado.*

I've always said, however, that there is a piece of this work that cannot be explained scientifically. It's what I call the "God Concept/God Component" or the "Universal Energy" or "Spirit" or that kind of thing. If IVF, for example, were simply a scientific process it would have a higher success rate—plain and simple. Especially now: they can control for so many variables, there are so many tests available, so many support drugs to ensure a healthy uterine lining, to balance hormones, etc.

But the medical community cannot control for the psychological component, they cannot control for the spiritual element. Subconscious blocks to fertility are my specialty— even a physiological impediment can have psychological roots. And there is a spiritual component here—not religious, though that can certainly be incorporated—but spiritual.

In his book, *The Biology of Belief,* Dr. Bruce Lipton (2005), a scientist and medical doctor straight out of what he likes to refer to as the "linear-minded," says that he now believes that Einstein and Newton ought to merge—that the world would benefit immensely from the acceptance of both quantum physics (considered right brain) and Newtonian (left brain) science. Dr. Lipton (2005) states that he was very happy to learn that scientists are unable to understand the secrets of the universe using linear thinking only.

Hyper-rational scientists, according to Lipton (2005) simply cannot offer the complete truth about the human body, let alone the universe. Though medical science continues to advance, says Lipton, we continue to find that living organisms pretty well refuse to be quantified. In other words, we have thus far been unable to glean indisputable scientific evidence with piecemeal examination of the world and its inhabitants—how can we hope to know the universe? We must realize the need for—and balance—left brain and right brain application. As my client base expanded across the globe I saw more and more of these spirit babies and had stronger and more detailed impressions. Eventually I began to share them with my clients and, to my surprise and delight, my clients were grateful for the input. I still wrestled with the process, especially because of Walter's work. I was quite happy with the arrangement: working his readings into my sessions whenever applicable.

I must add here, however, that there is one significant difference between Walter's work and mine: and that is unhappy spirit babies. I have NEVER—in tens of thousands of client hours—seen a spirit baby who is upset with any given situation. They are not subject to human attributes such as insecurity, fear, anger or vengefulness; they see—or perhaps more accurately, they *know*—the big picture. They are pure soul light; they are simply not limited as those of us in physical form are.

Dr. Brian Weiss, a Yale Medical School graduate and psychiatrist who is presently considered the leading expert on hypnotic past life regression worldwide, describes more than one level of learning for each of us. We learn some lessons in the flesh; we must feel. As a spirit, however, Dr. Weiss says we feel no pain (2000). He calls time spent in spirit a period of renewal because the soul is being renewed. We can (and do) feel pain in the physical state, in the flesh; we can hurt. Just as all my experience has indicated, in his book, *Messages from the Masters*, Dr. Weiss, too, states that we do not feel in spiritual form; there is only happiness, and a sense of well-being (2000). Since long before I began seeing the sparkly little orbs, or spirit babies, I have been leading clients through a process that connects them with their aborted, miscarried, stillborn or SIDS babies. These women (and sometimes men as well) have often been punishing themselves relentlessly for months, years, and even decades—though they may not always realize it—beating themselves up for something they don't even understand or could never have prevented. Often these traumas are untouched or unhealed in peoples' lives—whether they know it or not—and can become, or contribute to, the subconscious blocks that are preventing pregnancy.

Dr. Marion Woodman is a renowned Jungian psychologist, teacher and author who has literally decades of experience in her field. In her book, *The Pregnant Virgin,* Dr. Woodman shares some blatant insight regarding pregnancy, abortion and what I call "doing your own work." This information could apply to a client desiring to get pregnant or to her mother or grandmother. Sometimes when a woman comes to the threshold of separation from the mother, instead of taking the responsibility of birthing her own inner child she instead becomes obsessed with having a real baby (Woodman, 1985). The fear the woman has around her own inadequacies, and lack of identity cause her to desire to *be* someone—often the choice is to be a mother with an actual child onto whom she can project her own unresolved life.

Woodman says that if the woman is able to hold the tension until she finds herself—that is to say until she does her work—then if she does decide to have a baby, her baby will not have to carry what the woman, herself, fearfully avoided (Woodman, 1985). An abortion, says Woodman, can be the catalyst that forces a woman to strive to discover her own identity (1985). The baby in such case is the sacrifice through which the woman brings herself to birth. Bringing this to consciousness (as I have described above) and actually dealing with the issue *as* sacrifice—something of excessive value given up to something of even grander value—enables release of the underlying depression from the body and the psyche, creating balance and clarity.

I love this part of the HF process, I invite the babies to present themselves to their mothers and then I hold the silence while communion occurs. To see the smile of sheer joy spreading across my client's face as her baby shares divine knowing with her is, to me, a soul-felt gift. To bear witness to the dawning of an understanding that finally frees an anguished psyche is to gently tend a healing spirit. The babies are never angry and it reassures my clients to see for themselves. Often the baby(s) will soothe his/her mother, possibly even telling her that the baby is overseeing the coming of a daughter or son, or that the baby him/herself is coming back.

Over the years, world renown mediums and/or psychics such as George Anderson, James van Praagh, Sylvia Brown, Doreen Virtue, and others, have said publicly that "readings" often require interpretation of symbolism on the part of the reader, and that clarity, integrity, ego, beliefs, etc. can definitely have an impact on the discernment of information. I know that Walter has written and spoken of frightened spirit babies or spirit babies unhappy with their mother's choice of partner, etc. This is one subject that those who have spoken with Walter or read his book continually ask me about; they feel at fault or fear they will not conceive for this reason.

All I can say in that regard is to reiterate that I have never seen it. I personally believe, as do others I have consulted with, that everything is exactly as it needs to be, that miscarriages, abortions, divorces, etc. all have a place in the grand scheme of things and that these seemingly more human elements (judgment, anger, etc.) are exactly that—human impressions of Divine order. This statement is in no way meant to judge anyone else's work or interpretations, just to acknowledge that I have had questions in this regard, and this is the best way I can answer them.

Chapter 3

BABIES! BABIES!

"The most beautiful thing we can experience is the mysterious."

—*Albert Einstein*

Not long after I'd begun seeing the little spirit orb babies, but before I'd started to share the knowledge, a client of mine from about twelve years earlier came in for a Life Purpose Regression. She was not a fertility client; in fact, she came in for something completely unrelated. Since about 2002 my practice has been almost exclusively fertility clients but I do sometimes take referrals or will see former clients if they so desire. In this case I was seeing a client—Teri—who'd done quite a bit of work with me several years before but who was now dealing with a debilitating illness and wanted to do some hypnotic uncovering.

I proceeded to induce a deep level of hypnosis and then to regress Teri to what I call *The Between* so she could discover what, if any, spiritual contract had led to her ailment, and what she could do to heal. Teri's session was powerful and she was able to gain great insight from it. She had wanted to go straight to Source—to talk with God—and she did. As I began to wrap it up, Teri, still deep in hypnosis, stopped me and said, "They have a message for you."

"Who?" I asked her. At that Teri's face lit up and she spoke with awe: "Babies! Babies!" she exclaimed. "They LOVE you. They just LOVE you; they just want to BE with you. They want you to know that they are with you and they are happy that you help them find their parents but even if you didn't they still love to be with you!" Teri's face was an expression of pure bliss as she blurted out the words the spirit babies were asking her to share with me.

I must say that because of the work I do, and with all that I've seen over the years, I wasn't exactly surprised (if still a bit resistant) to have this happen during a client session. In fact, I was reminded of Dr. Brian Weiss's breakthrough book, *Many Lives, Many Masters,* where something similar happened to him during a patient session. In fact, Dr. Weiss's experience became the catalyst to his risking his distinguished psychiatric career to delve into—and eventually become the esteemed expert on—the world of hypnotic Past Life Regression.

As I said earlier, I do pay attention to what comes my way, so I accepted the message and pretty much declared to the Universe that I would take it forward, that I would open myself to the next level of this process however it needs to unfold. Within a couple of weeks of Teri's session and my rededication not only to HypnoFertility®, but to the entire *Spirit Baby Whisperer* process, I learned that Walter had died. On one level I was stunned, while on another level it made perfect sense to me.

I am sorry to say that Walter Makichen has, indeed, passed away. At the same time, I would like to take a moment to honor him and his contributions to the fertility world as we know it. Further information about his invaluable work can be found on his web site.

Chapter 4

SIGNS FROM THE BABIES

"The best way out is always through."

—*Robert Frost*

Back in 2005 I had evidence that there was an energy element that had to be considered in order for women to successfully become pregnant. Since my ability to envision it became clear a few years ago—and since I began to share the information with "my" babies' mothers, I have noticed a significant increase in pregnancies for my clients. I have come to realize, however, that my clients—these women and sometimes men or couples who come to work with me—are not really my clients. It's the babies who are actually my clients and if their parents need to see me these sparkly little cherubs see to it that their mommies "happen" to find me. When someone comes to see me, I know it is meant to be, I know what is behind the process.

I kept the knowledge of seeing spirit babies to myself initially—my left brain, my rational, analytical mind decided it was best. When this happens the spiritual world will find another way to reach out to you, and it will use what it knows you will believe or accept (eventually). I like very clear signs to occur in a sort of question and answer format. I knew what I was seeing could be called orbs because they appear to me as tiny, sparkly balls of light. I was telling this to my husband one day and I added something like *how am I going to find out more?*

The same day as this discussion, my husband Drake and I had to be way out in southeast Denver for a show our son Dylan was in. Finals were not until six hours after preliminaries so we had some time on our hands. We wandered around a newly built outdoor mall for a while. We came across a Barnes & Noble and both being avid readers decided to go in. As if I were being led by the hand I walked directly to the discount books area. I glanced around and then picked up a book by the psychic Sylvia Browne. I just popped it open to somewhere around the middle of the book and there, right in front of me, was a chapter on children's spirits and orbs.

I laughed and showed the book to my husband who looked at it (and me) with a what-did-you-expect grin. Of course, ask and ye shall receive. But just to make sure I was perfectly clear about what I was being shown, the Universe arranged for me to have an even clearer response to my orb question. I had flown to Chicago to teach a six-day HF and hypnosis/birthing intensive. A student in the class brought a book up to me on a break and said she thought I would like to see it. She was a very nice lady with a lovely turquoise aura that, in a pretty much completely white room, I could hardly miss noticing.

I had so much material to teach in such little time that the book sat up on the platform behind me for days without me getting a chance to look at it. On the last day of training my colleague, at whose school I was teaching, was slotted to teach an afternoon segment of about an hour. As it began I realized I could finally look at the book and none too soon as Joni, the student who had brought the book, had to leave immediately at the end of the training. I took a seat toward the back of the room and proceeded to open the book—as I always do, to somewhere around the middle or wherever it falls open to— and this time there was a photo of a whole bunch of orbs, my orbs, just like I'd been seeing. And under a heading: *Orbs Are People Too!*

The book was called *The Children of Now* and I really wanted to read it. I decided to order it from Amazon.com, wondering how long that would take, all the while trying to absorb as much as I could before I had to resume teaching. At the break Joni was happy to see that I'd looked at the book. I thanked her for bringing it and told her that the photo of the orbs looked just like the ones I see in my office. At that, she gave me the book and insisted I read it on the plane. She said she felt that Spirit wanted me to have it so I accepted it with deep gratitude and appreciation.

I often recommend *The Children of Now* to clients and students. Not only did the orb photo match my visual perceptions of the spirit babies, but a good deal of the material the author has gathered on the children fits within the *Spirit Baby Whisperer* paradigm that was evolving within my awareness. I like spiritual author Doreen Virtue's writings about the Indigo, Crystal, and Rainbow Children as well. The *Spirit Baby Whisperer* information came to me through my own spiritual cognizance and sentience; the visuals simply appeared. I had never heard of these other works prior to my own energetic evolution; it was interesting to see some of what the babies were showing and telling me also in print.

Dr. Meg Blackburn Losey (2007), author of *The Children of Now*, shines some light onto the various types of children and their reason for being. She says the Indigo Children are the paradigm busters who inherently know that something is wrong in our world. The Indigos know that the rules of society do not necessarily consider the particular circumstances of—or the individuals in—any given situation. The Indigos, in creating awareness, have opened doors for human kind to recognize and nurture future generations.

Dr. Doreen Virtue (2012) says that both Indigo Children (born over the past 100 years) and Crystal Children (born since around the 1990s) are the next step in our evolution as human beings, who are here to show us the way. Indigos continued to be born until around 2000 with increasing abilities and levels of technological and creative sophistication. Crystals, says Virtue (2012) are a powerful force for peace and love on our planet. Both highly sensitive and psychic, Crystal Children tend to be even-tempered or even blissful while Indigos have the warrior spirit necessary for their collective life purpose of dismantling what no longer works. The Indigos are tough so the Crystals don't have to be.

"There are greater realities just beyond most people's perception" (Losey, 2007). Dr. Losey stresses that it is important to be aware that there are infinite dimensions throughout all of creation, and those dimensions are part of the concept of the One—that which is known as God, Spirit, or the Creator—and there are infinite possibilities within these realities. Each being is created of layers of subtle energy; that energy communicates outwardly, inwardly, and infinitely with all other levels of reality.

Particularly pertinent to the spirit babies, to the sparkly little orbs who guide their mothers to see me, is the validation of that which they have been trying to convey to my clients—to you—in one way or another. According to Losey (2007) it used to be that we quickly forgot our true origin upon the birth of the physical body. We would forget (or deeply bury) our Source, our gifts, our perfection. The spirit babies, the babies who are coming through now, both remember and embody that which we have forgotten. As such there truly is the opportunity for positive change in our world.

The knowledge the spirit babies have imparted to me over the past few years is reiterated by Losey (2007) and what she has received from her *Children of Now*. There is more to our reality than we may presently know or accept but in order to bring them through we must listen intently to the spirit babies and open ourselves to what they are saying. These little light beings have important messages for us and are a powerful Source energy connection. "The children are here and they are now—and there are more on the way!" (Losey, 2007). Are you open to the process?

Chapter 5

THE FIRST HYPNOFERTILITY® BABY

"It is the nature of babies to be in bliss."

—*Deepak Chopra*

Lynsi:

My son, Dylan, calls himself the first HypnoFertility®
Baby. He certainly is for me, officially at least. Dylan taught me
the process with which I have been working all these years. It
is because of him that I know that all of this is absolutely true,
and that I can work with my clients—those who resonate with
me—so confidently. Dylan has agreed to tell his half of our
story here in this book; to speak to you from where your
babies are now. He is just shy of 18-years-old at this writing
and he and I have been communicating about this since before
he was conceived. He wants to share it with you; he truly cares
about your wellbeing and the importance of the spirit baby
connection.

I will start with my version and will have to back up a
bit first. My oldest son, Kelly, was conceived at a tumultuous
time. His 32-year-old uncle had just been killed in a terrible
head on collision with a tractor trailer (I'd had to identify the

body), and two months later my father (age 50) had died suddenly of a massive coronary. He died in my arms as I tried all I could do to save him. Kelly, conceived between these two traumatizing events, was doused in cortisol (a tiny 6-week fetus) as fight or flight took charge of me and I willed my body and my brain to keep my father alive. It was not to be.

I did manage to keep Kelly alive, however, and thus began my adult journey into the realm of mind/body/spirit balance. My father's heart attack had been caused by stress it was determined, and that was really not surprising knowing all that had been going on in his life at the time of his death, and knowing that he had survived (or perhaps escaped would be more accurate) a seriously abusive childhood that had laid the groundwork for his early demise. From a hypnotic standpoint, this is called reinforcement or compounding. I'll discuss that more a little later.

I have naturally utilized hypnotic ability since I was a child. I didn't realize it at the time, of course, but it is easy now to see why I would be drawn to it as one of the most powerful tools possible for spirit baby whispering. My beautiful baby son was born on the 5th of September, 1989, at barely 36 weeks. The doctor was incompetent (I won't go into it) and I thought I was going to lose him too for a little while. My mind actually shut down at this point and I basically left my body. Then, somehow, Kelly was alright but they were whisking him off to the NICU. This was at the hospital where the ambulance had taken my father six months earlier. Trauma number three for me in less than one year.

I decided I didn't want any more children and before Kelly was four months old his father had a vasectomy. I was 21-years-old; people questioned me and I just said, "If God wants me to have another baby I will." (I was not religious.) Kelly has an older half-brother, Coady, and half-sister, Candace, so I felt he would have siblings regardless.

Fast forward to 1993: I suddenly became aware of . . . it was hard to put words to it at the time. But, eventually I figured it out and I told my (ex)husband that I felt like there was a baby there, that we should have another baby. He asked what I wanted to do about it and eventually we decided to see a doctor about reversing the vasectomy. They told us chances were slim to none. I simply declared, "If I'm supposed to have another baby I will, if not, it's not meant to be." We scheduled the surgery in June of 1993.

By the time we had the all-clear from the surgery we had learned we were being transferred to Lawrenceville, GA (from Kitchener, ON). We put any thoughts of babies on hold and put our house on the market. By November 1993 we were living in Georgia, but I had no work visa and things were pretty much up in the air. I knew the baby was there but it just wasn't time. I began working with hypnosis and meditation in a more official capacity and doing guided journeys every day. One day in May of 1994 I just knew it was time. By the first weekend in June I had a confirmed pregnancy. By then I was already certain that I would have another baby but the physical pregnancy confirmation seems to make it more real for most people.

I visited my baby throughout the pregnancy; I would go and "hang out" with him through the hypnotic process. The doctors told me he was a girl and everyone kept saying that. I just didn't think so. (Neither did Kelly; in fact, he'd insisted from the beginning that the baby was a boy.) One day I got his name: Dylan James. I told his dad and his dad said that the baby is a girl so we don't need a boy's name. I basically said okay but if it's a boy can we name him Dylan James? He said yes, thinking I was off my rocker no doubt. Well, you already know how this turns out: January 18th, 1995, Dylan James.

My sweet little Dylan was a happy baby, just like his older brother had been. When Kelly was three he used to freak out his babysitter by talking about where he *used* to be. I asked him where he used to be one day after she'd mentioned it and he said, "At the light."

"Well, of course, at the light," I'd thought chuckling. Kelly used to always tell me about knowing and being with his Grandpa Garry (my father). My spiritual instructor told me to test Kelly's sensitivity by having him guess playing cards: red and black. Kelly could usually get more than 30 right which is considered quite good. I started using a little kid's *Go Fish* deck and he could get nearly all of those cards. Not red/black either, but goldfish, starfish, dolphin, whatever the picture was.

As Dylan began to talk he spoke of the light too. But he also spoke of how he had picked me, how he had wanted me for his mommy, how he'd told me he was coming, and how I had listened. He told me that he had wanted his name and that he had wanted to be a boy. He said that babies pick their parents and the parents are supposed to listen for them. He told me the same thing over and over for years; in fact, he still says the same things.

Just as Dylan has always said, Dr. Brian Weiss (2000) also tells us that we choose our parents, and that usually these are souls we have interacted with in prior lifetimes. Dr. Weiss reminds us that upon entering the physical realm we learn, first as children, then as adolescents, and finally as adults; we evolve spiritually even as our bodies evolve physically. And though we often forget this we do know on some level that any seemingly negative event in our lives may well be a door opening to a much better opportunity. Your destiny is unfolding every day; destiny sometimes just needs time to weave its intricate tapestry.

Dylan is a Sensitive—more about that later. He is what is called a Crystal Child, as I mentioned in the last chapter—he is here to help heal the planet. The children of my clients are Crystals and now what are being called Rainbow Children. This is why there is a greater need than ever to help them through from spirit to physical. Or, maybe it is better said that they are helping us to help them through.

According to Doreen Virtue (2010) the first thing many people notice about Crystal Children is their eyes—they have large, penetrating eyes that are clearly wise beyond their years. These happy, delightful, forgiving little sweeties are capable of seeing straight through to your soul, and are unlike any previous generation of lightworkers. Crystal Children are blissful and even-tempered, forgiving and easy-going for the most part. The Crystals are the generation meant to benefit from the trailblazing of the Indigos.

The Indigo Children, with their warrior spirits, are the pioneers of the lightworkers, in most cases generations ahead of the Crystals and Rainbows. The Indigos blazed the trail with a machete—ripping down everything without integrity—enabling the Crystal Children to follow the cleared path into a more secure, safer world. Indigos share some characteristics with the Crystal Children (Virtue, 2010). Both are highly sensitive and psychic; and both have vital life purposes. The difference between them is basically their temperament. Indigos came through first to pave the way for Crystals and Rainbows, to use their fiery dispositions and unwavering strength to get rid of antiquated systems interfering with the overall integrity of the planet.

The Rainbow Children, often referred to as fearless, are just beginning to arrive (Virtue, 2010) and are the temperament of many of the incoming spirit babies. They are pure givers ready to fulfill our needs; the embodiment of divinity and the example of our potential. The little Rainbows are all about service; they are here simply to give. Rainbow Children, according to Doreen Virtue (2010), have already reached their spiritual peak. It is for this reason—the shifting of the planetary energies due to increased spiritual vibration—that the spirit babies are seeking help with alignment.

Dylan has always said to me, "Thank you, Mom, for giving me life." He says it out of the blue, and especially when he was very little I would be awed by the statement. From a five-o'clock-world standpoint (what I call the more mainstream society) I have no idea where he got that—I've never given him the: *You're lucky to be alive, I went through X hours of labor because of you . . .* guilt trip speech. From the *Spirit Baby Whisperer* world view this is just one more expression of Dylan's Crystal qualities.

When Dylan was four he would tell me what was wrong with my pediatric clients. At one time I was seeing a lot of four and five-year-olds and without telling Dylan anything about them he would tell me what they were afraid of or what was going on. I'd tuck what he said in the back of my mind and sure enough he would be right. He does this now, he'll

45

walk through the room where I do my Skype calls and off handedly mention that whatever client I've just spoken to is going to have a girl or some information of a similar sort.

A few years ago for my birthday Dylan got me a bamboo plant in an elephant pot. He didn't know what it meant, he was just drawn to it and felt I should have it. I looked up Feng Shui and elephant and found that the elephant is for fertility. (Of course!) I asked Dylan if I could take the bamboo to my office where I felt it would do a lot of good and he agreed. It is often the topic of conversation, particularly when new clients come in. I can't count how many people have told me they were just immediately drawn to it when they walked in—they like to hear the story, and they like Dylan's involvement. He is often seen by my clients as an energetic spirit baby bridge, and they can feel his energy emanating from that incredible little plant.

Dylan:

I just started by picking my mom. I don't really remember much about that part, all I know is I chose her. I was drawn to my name and drawn to my mom and so here I am. You don't choose the spirit baby the spirit baby chooses you. A lot of the times, in cases of infertility, it has more to do with your open-mindedness and attraction to the spirit babies than it does with an actual problem. If you pick a name before you know you are pregnant it will help, it kind of gives the spirit baby an anchor. My mom knew my name subconsciously even though it seems I gave it to her. I did give it to her yet she already knew because we're so connected.

A spirit baby is an incomplete entity, it needs a mother. It's not that you can or can't function as a spirit baby, just not at one hundred per cent. It is up to the mother to appeal to the spirit baby, but remember, spirit babies have different personalities just like we do. My mom stood out to me, appealed to me and my needs, so I chose to be born to her. Everyone's life purpose is to live and to learn. My focus is music—to me it is an entire rainbow of emotions. The point is not so much what my life purpose is but how I live my life purpose. That's the same for everyone, including the spirit babies.

There are different groupings, infinite numbers of spirit babies, constantly being created and recreated, being born, attracted to every person. The same group of spirit babies may recycle, may be reborn into the same family: grandfathers, grandmothers, brothers, aunts, miscarried or aborted babies, etc. We cycle through the infinite 8. By that I mean the infinity symbol—like an 8 laying on its side—if you can imagine tracing the 8 over and over, that's what I mean. If the spirit baby changes they get sucked into a different 8.

A lot of attracting your spirit baby is about knowing your true self—not necessarily understanding yourself but knowing. And being open-minded is important. My mom refers to it as being in balance and being receptive. You could say that my mom is easy to see for the spirit babies, just like she was for me. That's why it's easy for her to help them to connect with their moms.

Dylan dictated his piece to me as though he were speaking directly to you—I simply keyed it into the computer as he was speaking and cleaned up the grammar and punctuation later.

Chapter 6

SPIRIT BABY MAMA

"People are like stained-glass windows.
They sparkle and shine when the sun is out, but when the darkness sets
in, their true beauty is revealed only if there is a light from within."

—*Elizabeth Kübler-Ross*

A few days before the Spring Equinox, Dylan asked me if we could go to the mountains together for a day or two. We are both earth signs so grounding is especially essential to us, and we are quite in tune with the necessity. I asked where he wanted to go and he immediately told me Glenwood Springs. Glenwood Springs, Colorado is an incredible healing mecca that, like other faraway spiritual places such as Machu Picchu, draws in souls in search of deep spiritual and physical restoration from around the world. A sacred sulphured hot spring nestled beneath the starry mountain skies affords the panoramic view of snowy mountain slopes and—courtesy of the bright, golden aspens and colossal evergreens—crisp, fresh air tousles the hair, soothes the skin, and rejuvenates the breath.

Symbolically, energetically, the awareness that where such extraordinary healing waters are found imparts the knowledge that as underground shifting—the source of the burbling waters—occurs and continues the earth is not only very much alive but still growing, and the absorption of rejuvenating, renewing, creative, fertile energies occurs without effort. The three natural elements: earth, air, and water are impeccably balanced as well, reinforcing the healing process on all levels. Earth represents the physical: the physical body, the physical/material world. Air is the mind, the brain, the intellect. Water is emotion, intuition, the psyche, the spirit. I am well aware that we are privileged to be able to visit the Springs virtually anytime via a gorgeous drive of only a couple of hours up, around, and through the depths of the mountain canyons, immersed in the richness of the Earth Mother herself.

Both our schedules were tight so our plan was to drive up, check into our hotel, and go right to the hot spring pools which are open until 10 p.m. Dylan and I are both night owls so that was actually quite appealing to us. The pools are much less crowded during the evening hours which makes it easier to relax, and easier to meditate. There is a saying: *healer, heal thyself.* It is a true statement and it is essential; you will often hear me talking about self-care which is applicable to both clients and therapists always.

It is during such times of my own self-care that I will receive new information or that ideas will come to me. This time was to be no different though the energetic signature in the hot springs that night was heightened: the combination of HF mom and original HF baby. The March night air still held the bite of winter as Dylan and I made our way toward the steaming water. We slipped in quickly, right up to our necks, and without a word we both laid our heads back and drifted into meditation.

Many years ago I learned a hypnosis technique designed to take you into what I call *The Between.* Life purpose regressions, past life regressions, hypnotic gestalt, and spirit baby whisperings tend to make use of *The Between.* There are many names for *The Between*: the invisible world, the other side, the beyond, the light, the mist, etc. In this particular journey there is a doorway that leads to a version of *The Between* that is a type of angel or fairy city, town or village. There are gardens, carnivals and many buildings; once, in my meanderings, I even came across an angelic fertility clinic. I quite like it here, the lights and colors are brilliant yet peaceful and the vibrations are fast and high, just as one would expect to encounter with angels or other beings of light.

I didn't have any meditation in particular in mind as the hot sulphur water and minerals sluiced over me and I began to relax; before my eyes were barely closed, however, I was at the golden doorway, entering the splendid garden of light, and retrieving my key from beneath a drop of rainwater glistening on the petal of one of my favorite roses, vibrant and purple. I unlocked the gate and proceeded to wander about the little village knowing I was welcome and wanted. I became aware of a magnetic-like force drawing me toward the city center so I relaxed into it and let go.

In a blink I was on the steps leading into the Universal Fertility Clinic; it's actually more like a spa. I was inside, in the lobby; then I was in a nursery-like room filled with spirit babies. Intuitively, telepathically, I somehow heard or experienced the word "mama." It was coming from all the little sparkly babies, as were the sensations of unconditional love and pure bliss that enveloped me instantly like an exquisite cloak of brilliant light.

In what resembled an instant (computer) download I received the information that I am "mama" to the spirit babies, that many of them stick in my aura and accompany me to speaking engagements, teaching dates, and to private HF sessions. I understood that the psychic information would continue to get stronger and that I needed to tell my clients about it. Also, that the HF work is necessary, that the psychic information will not be enough to bring babies through, and that the combination of both would be unprecedented. From this instantaneous transmission I learned that I am to write and publish the book explaining the spirit babies' alignment plight, and was assured that only the parents I am to help will be drawn to me. Meditate, listen, trust ended the communication and reminded me of the essentials I am to teach others, and what I am to honor myself.

My eyes opened and I found myself gazing up into a velvety indigo sky intricately patterned with stars of fiery white crystal ice; shimmering silver. This spectacular view caused me to wonder for a moment if my meditation had actually ended or not, but the crisp night air and steamy water quickly refocused me. Continuing to soak I reflected on this latest spirit baby initiated communication, and what it meant both for me and my clients. Destinies written in the stars I mused as I gazed upward in complete alignment, in complete balance, and in harmony mind, body, and spirit.

Walter Makichen (Spirit Babies, 2005) is told by a little girl spirit baby he meets in a sacred wooded area that there are places called joining places where it is easier for spirit babies to pass through from the spirit world to the physical. He asks her if there are other spirits like her waiting for their parents in the actual place where their conversation is occurring. Her response is yes, but she also says that some have no parents and are in need of a mother and father. In these cases they wait in joining places and/or with joining people.

My Glenwood Springs meditation was yet another reinforcement of what the spirit babies had communicated to me in so many ways over so many years. It reinforced what the little spirit baby girl had told Walter on that fateful day as well. Similarly, according to Dr. Brian Weiss (2001) before we are born we help set up and arrange learning opportunities and destiny points in our lives. Divine, spiritual energies help us to devise our lesson plans, and sometimes we may notice feelings of déjà vu. These are actually a dim remembering of our pre-natal plan as it is activated in the physical state right at the designated time and place during our unfolding lives.

I had not necessarily expected the specific meditation experience to occur, though I wasn't surprised either. I had already encountered this same type of spirit baby or energetic expression, communication, and connection during client sessions, in readings over the years, and—according to my friend and gifted astrologer, Karen Anderson—my entire natal chart depicts exactly what is unfolding; such is my destiny.

Chapter 7

EMANATING INDIGO

*"We grow primarily through our challenges,
especially those life-changing moments when we begin to recognize aspects of
our nature that make us different from the family and
culture in which we have been raised."*

—*Caroline Myss*

One afternoon in early 2009 I was working with a client, we'll call her Sophie, at my office. This was a client I particularly enjoyed working with as she was very dedicated to her process. Not only did she want to become pregnant but she wanted to be sure she had healed from her own childhood trauma so that she could be a truly good mother.

As Sophie was talking that day I became aware of a dark blue tinge covering her upper right arm from the shoulder to the elbow. It was very apparent to me and no matter how she moved or what I did this indigo light remained. I jotted a note to myself to look this phenomenon up later that night. I knew it was aura related; I'd taken aura reading classes as part of energy work I'd done years earlier. I'd even taught others how to read them. But now I recalled my very first spiritual teacher, Homer, from decades ago, back in Kitchener, Ontario.

Homer had been able not only to see auras but to read them, and he had taught his students that every body part represented something as did the various colors.

When I got home I got on the internet and proceeded to research "indigo arm." I also tried blue, blue light, blue aura, blue light on arm, and every other combination of possibilities I could think of. All I kept bumping into was "Indigo Children" and that was a subject I had always avoided. Until now. I finally gave in and decided to read the information on Indigo Children. My only past experience with this subject was extremist groups using the term to disguise bad parenting: *my child doesn't follow direction because he's an Indigo, my child pulls all the other children's hair at school because she's an Indigo, my child can only eat at McDonald's because she's an Indigo*, and that type of thing.

I just thought that kind of thinking was ridiculous and I didn't want to have anything to do with it. But Sophie's Indigo display opened a whole new world for me. Upon reading the material I learned what Indigo Children really are, and that they have been followed to this physical world by Crystal and Rainbow Children. I learned that I, myself, am an Indigo Child/Adult, and that there is a very obvious reason for that given my life purpose as the *Spirit Baby Whisperer*.

I have been telling my clients for several years now that they have been specifically chosen to undergo this infertility experience so that they may become the vessels for highly sensitive, gifted children to enter the physical world. I received this information from the babies and from God via claircognizant communication, often through meditation. There is a reason that not just anyone comes to me as a client, and it is my understanding that the ones who do are guided to me by their very own babies.

Dr. Brian Weiss (2001) says that the raising of children must be altered, particularly the raising of boys. There is no reason why boys should not be raised to be aware of and to express more sensitivity. Teaching girls to have more confidence and to be more self-assertive is important too, but because the violence in the world today is caused almost exclusively by men, the reason for the energy shift with incoming babies becomes quite apparent. I was blessed with boys and I did raise them to have heightened sensitivity—it is virtually palpable in them. The planet needs this from you and your children as well.

I said in *It's Conceivable!* that I began to pay attention early on when my clients told me that they just knew there was a baby there. And then they became pregnant despite doctors giving them a zero per cent chance or other such grim prognoses. Tens of thousands of clinic hours since the early days have confirmed what I intuited to be true even then—that the parent/baby connection, the God-concept as I often call it—is stronger than any man-made construct. If you feel there is a baby there I believe you.

As I mentioned earlier I am what is called an Indigo Adult. Basically, that is a grown up Indigo Child. There are different views on how long the Indigos have been around but for the past 100 years is common among sources. To expand a bit on what I discussed in Chapter 5, the early Indigos were called scouts; they came to pave the way for the next wave. I was born in the sixties while what are considered the "pure" Indigos weren't born until the eighties. Indigo children were quite rare when I was a child, and they were not particularly popular.

Indigos tend to be considered creative rebels, nonconformists who have a heightened sensitivity to the energies of others. I had a very difficult time as a child but that is to be expected as an Indigo. I can see now that my childhood had to be that challenging so that I could develop the right skills to properly express my life purpose. Indigos are born with a warrior spirit and they often encounter tough times early on so that they can strengthen it.

I wasn't bad—just different; and smarter than a number of the adults around me (not to mention the kids) so I often challenged their beliefs, though not necessarily intentionally. I just wanted to know why. I could easily see when people were lying, and I could feel their emotional pain. In elementary and middle school I was a loner for the most part, and I have been a vegetarian pretty much since birth.

Sometimes I think I made it tough on myself because I wouldn't conform; I wouldn't follow a bunch of girls around, and I wouldn't lead them.

I was very much alone as an Indigo Child but now I run into other Indigos quite often. They are attracted to the healing fields so I meet Indigo therapists, and, I believe because of something the spirit babies need, I often have Indigo clients. The life purpose of Indigos, as I mentioned earlier, is to quash old systems, dismantle or break down and get rid of what no longer works. My little piece of the Indigo purpose is to do that with fertility. The ways of invasive, emotionally trying, ultra-expensive treatments are out of balance. It's not that they're not helpful, but they need to be done in a more holistic manner.

I need my Indigo qualities so that I can hold the emotional space with clients, and understand and validate the things they have been through without judgment. As a pioneer in this field, and the creator of the first class ever to teach other therapists, I have had to deal with a few things: some men in the field initially dismissing the work as if it were an insignificant hobby, professional jealousy, slander, harassment, and theft. Nothing that isn't to be expected should one find oneself in the trailblazer position—and that's exactly why I can see the need for my Indigo assets. I am grateful to have them and I wouldn't change a thing—past, present or future.

As an Indigo I am able to see and read the energy of clients and spirit babies and therefore facilitate the desired connection. My Indigo sensitivity easily engages the spirit babies' Crystal and Rainbow energies and makes it easy for them to communicate with me, as though I am a bridge between the physical world and Source. I am strong enough to be a voice for this important work, and because I have no need to be like anybody else I can speak from authenticity, honesty, and truth. I am dedicated to my life purpose and the Universe has made sure to provide me with every single thing I need. And thus, I find myself the *Spirit Baby Whisperer*.

Chapter 8

SENSITIVES

"I saw the angel in the marble and carved until I set him free."

—*Michelangelo*

I have often been described as an Empath, a Sensitive, or Ultra-Sensitive. I once bought a book because it was entitled *Are You Really Too Sensitive?* I had certainly been told so my entire life. A sensitive is able to read the feelings of others from a somewhat magnified perspective. It is often when this occurs that the other person accuses you of being too sensitive or too sensitive for your own good (because you hit on something they don't want to address or even acknowledge). Actually, according to the author of the above mentioned book, Marcy Calhoun, "you are just as sensitive as you are supposed to be" (1987).

Everyone is sensitive to some extent, but there are those who are sensitive to the extent that others become very aware of it. People are most often uncomfortable with anything that is in the least bit different to what they consider to be normal. After years of doing the work I do I find myself unable to say the words "normal" or "reality" without air quotes, but that's just me. When help is needed, however—when healing is desired desperately—people tend to relinquish their more conservative ideas and open themselves to the world that Sensitives have always known.

In the case of spirit babies, that is a necessary shift as the incoming children are exactly that: sensitive. Highly sensitive. Because of the sweetness, because of the gentleness of what are being referred to now as Rainbow Children, they need parents who will honor their emotional delicateness by providing an environment conducive to such kind little personalities. The Indigo and Crystal Children are Sensitives too, however not to the extent of the Rainbows. Doreen Virtue is considered to be one of the top experts on these children. The Rainbows, she says, are "the embodiment of our divinity, and the example of our potential" (2010).

Sensitives are not necessarily Indigo, Crystal, or Rainbow but for our spirit baby intents and purposes these are what we will largely be dealing with. The Crystals, as I mentioned earlier, are born mostly between the early nineties and the present, and are wise beyond their years, happy, loving, and forgiving (Virtue, 2010). The Indigos are highly sensitive but with a warrior spirit and firey determination. The earliest Indigos, known as scouts, often chose abusive or difficult homes to grow up in as part of their purpose: leading the way; mashing down old systems, systems without integrity, or those that no longer serve us.

As you know, I am an Indigo Adult; it makes perfect sense that I should be when I look at my life purpose. Bringing babies into this world from an energetic/spiritual standpoint is not exactly how we've been doing it (at least knowingly) since the beginning of human existence. I grew up in a way that would toughen me up, that would prepare me to challenge the rules, to break from the herd, and to not just go along to get along. I was sensitive enough to be open to this work right from the start, and determined enough to get it out there. I don't really care what anyone else thinks so nothing could deter me.

Empaths are able to sense others on many levels. They are able to read energy patterns or vibrations, and have a "knowing" with regard to the feelings and needs of others. Empaths are often described as sensitive, and sometimes the terms are used interchangeably. Empaths are highly intuitive and they are excellent listeners. You'll often find Empaths in the worlds of therapy, healing, and the arts as these are perfect venues for their specific skills.

Empaths must learn to shield, that is to say they must learn how not to take on too much of other people's "stuff." An Empath is able to empathize with a client, to quickly and effectively understand where that client is coming from. The Empath must be in balance, however, or their information will be skewed. Sometimes it is difficult for an Empath to tell their own "stuff" from that of others. For this reason many Empaths and Sensitives choose to avoid large crowds; when they have to be at the airport, for example, they often find themselves feeling very drained very quickly.

I teach my clients energetic shielding mainly because it is essential as far as spirit baby and mother vibration alignment. Also, my clients tend to be subjected to a lot of negativity and that will keep knocking them off balance if we don't address it. I have a number of ways to create and utilize powerful shielding mechanisms, and they reinforce any and all other work I do with my clients. Shielding is certainly beneficial to non-sensitive people; however, the spirit babies are Sensitives and a great number of my clients "happen" to fall into one of the above categories as well.

Knowing all this ahead of time enables you not only to get pregnant, but also to prepare for a peaceful pregnancy and a gentle birth experience. HF babies are known for their calmness (after all, they respond to the hypnosis too). Mothers are pleased to tell me that they had a quick, easy recovery (c-section or vaginal birth), and that nursing went even more smoothly than expected. So, in other words, pre-conception your baby benefits from your shielding; post-conception—throughout your pregnancy—post-natal and beyond, you'll find your baby benefits from it as well.

Chapter 9

A VESSEL FOR YOUR BABY

"It is in your moments of decision that your destiny is shaped."

—*Tony Robbins*

An issue I've found myself dealing with more and more frequently is donor eggs. This has always been a touchy subject and understandably so. Years ago it wasn't as common and most of my clients were focused on natural conception or IVF. At that time FSH (Follicle Stimulating Hormone) was the hot topic; now it's low ovarian reserve or AMH (Anti-Mullerian Hormone) and donor eggs. Interestingly, my clients have shifted from an average age of about 41 to an average age of about 44.

I have done a lot of what I call damage control around this subject. There is a local clinic that is well known for "pushing" donor eggs; in fact, I can guess what clinic someone has been to based on the way donor eggs were recommended to them. Clients are always amazed when I say, "Oh, you went to X clinic."

Donor eggs may look like the best choice from a scientific and detached standpoint, however, women (couples) are human beings and the emotional impact of diagnosis and

61

prognosis must be considered to avoid traumatizing the people involved. The trauma of being told that donor eggs are virtually the only option can slice through the subconscious mind like a dagger, imbedding itself there in the form of a subconscious block, and inhibiting successful pregnancy, donor egg or otherwise.

Some women have no issue with donor eggs; others struggle for months or even years with the concept. Single women in their mid to late 40s are pretty much limited to that option if they want to be pregnant: donor eggs and donor sperm. I still work with those women to be receptive to the embryos even if they had no difficulty coming to their decision. I spend more time with women who need to come to terms with donor eggs, to grieve the loss of using their own eggs, and to be receptive to the donor egg embryos at transfer.

Women need to decide on donor eggs (if they make that decision) in their own time. I tell my clients that this is their process and they can't compare it to anyone else's process. Some need to scream and cry; others need to retreat or withdraw for a while. Some women need to talk it over with their partners many times, while some need to go to support groups. Some need to tell all their friends, and some need to keep it to themselves. The point here is that whatever your process is you need to honor it, and allow it to unfold.

Some women never get to donor eggs; they decide they'd prefer to remain childless, to adopt, to continue to try naturally, to go ahead with IVF using their own eggs at another clinic. This is where the balance comes in, where in the silence of your mind you can hear your intuition, hear the messages from your baby(s), and know what to do. This is what we are working toward with HF. Whether or not you're going to do donor is not the issue; you knowing from a place of internal certainty what is right for you and your baby _is_.

Gavin de Becker, author of _The Gift of Fear_, explains that what others may try to dismiss as just a gut feeling or a coincidence actually is a cognitive process that is much faster than we recognize and very different than process or step-by-step thinking that we rely upon so typically, so easily, and so willingly (1997). de Becker confirms what I have been teaching clients and students for decades: though we have been taught to think that conscious thought is better, intuition is, in fact, lightning-fast compared to the quicksand-like actions of logic. Intuition is A to Z without stopping for any other letter. Intuition is knowing even if we don't know why.

I have always cautioned my clients that fear masquerades as intuition. If you are out of balance you will not be able to discern what it is that you need to hear. Discounting your intuition is a sure way to weaken it, and to make room for fear to invade and conquer. The Universe gave me a clear example of the very issue a few years ago: I was walking my dogs (approximately 70 lbs each with pit bullish features) in a nature reserve late one night without my husband. Suddenly I became aware that a stalker—most likely Jason from the horror movie *Friday the 13th*—was hiding behind the trees, waiting to jump out at me.

I rationalized that the dogs weren't growling or barking or even paying any attention, and that Jason is just a character from a stupid movie. My "intuition" (which I knew to be fear) screamed that this was not so, that I was about to be killed. I was laughing (though also a bit creeped out) because I knew exactly what the Universe was demonstrating; and that it was giving me a good story to share with clients. I know how to sense into my intuition and tell if it is authentic or fear; but for those who haven't yet cultivated that skill fear can take right over. Intuition is essential; fear is detrimental. Fear puts you through unnecessary stress and takes a toll on your physiology; on your entire mind, body, spirit balance.

Thinking back through your life, you can probably recall at least one incident where you heeded your intuition and were so relieved you did. Each of us has intuition, we simply must develop it. To do that, we must first acknowledge it, which is easier to do when we utilize a bit of hindsight: intuition heeded. According to de Becker (1997), intuition is far more valuable than plain knowledge. We tend to value hindsight over foresight—and paying attention to hindsight can help us streamline foresight—but heeded intuition (hindsight) is the key to learning how to trust your intuition exclusively and without a doubt. So you will be confident in your decision-making anytime you need to be.

The babies don't care what you decide. And, basically, what you decide is exactly what is supposed to be anyway. Your baby is with you already. In spirit. In energy form. You can feel your baby's presence. The embryo—the egg and sperm—that is just the body. Your baby joins the body when one is available. Your baby is your baby and wants you to know that you don't have to doubt it. Yes, you will love him/her—your baby is your baby. Again, natural, IVF, donor, adoption or otherwise—your baby is your baby. Donor eggs are simply a vehicle, a vessel for your baby.

Chapter 10

LIVING MY DHARMA

*"Your work is to discover your world and then with all your heart
give yourself to it."*

—Buddha

One of my clients recently pointed out that I am
"living my dharma." In other words, I'm doing what I was put
on earth for, following my path. She is absolutely right. And in
following my path I assist others in following theirs: becoming
parents to sensitive little beings who have contracted with
them for a shared purpose, for reasons of self-growth,
spirituality, and healing the planet.

We all have a life purpose; we chose it before we ever
came into this physical world. But the density of the energies
here often makes it difficult for us to remember our purpose.
We may have a sense, an inkling of sorts; we may follow
hunches without realizing they are really spiritual guidance. We
do tend to encounter the right people at the right times; as the
Buddha says, "When the student is ready, the teacher will
appear." But we have to be awake and paying attention in
order to progress to the next level.

The Creator has a way of nudging me along that is unique to my personality. When I am about to reach the next level with my spiritual growth the Creator places a choice before me that actually allows me to move energy. Not long before I published *It's Conceivable!* I was pondering whether or not I should publish it. I suddenly found myself the co-creator of an in-great-demand weight loss program that was sweeping Colorado.

I was putting in at least eighty hours per week between the fertility work and the weight loss program. The weight loss program was quite lucrative and had excellent franchise appeal. I ran with both for some time but then realized I was becoming quite drained from working with the weight loss clients. Most were not willing to take responsibility for their issues, and wanted my partner and me to do everything for them. Our program worked wonders for these people, but all in all we were both feeling incredibly drained.

I realized that for as drained as I was by the weight clients, I was easily as equally energized by my fertility clients. These clients are highly motivated, they want to have a baby, and they are willing to "do the work" or participate in the process, if you will. Before I knew it I had crystal clear awareness that I needed to dissolve the weight loss company and publish *It's Conceivable!* You can tell when you've made the right choice because everything goes so smoothly.

Within weeks of the release of my book, and my first book signing at a conference on a Caribbean cruise, I had interviews by ABC, CBS, half a dozen magazines and a radio interview in Australia, television appearances on Toronto's *Breakfast Television* and Canada's *At Home Show*, and more. I appeared briefly on the eleven o'clock news in Los Angeles which resulted in clients flocking in from California, and the need for me to schedule an emergency LA therapist training to handle the requests for therapists trained in my methods. We had to turn people away from that training.

On top of all that, during my whirlwind trip to the Los Angeles area I also managed to squeeze in a couple of hours to give a talk at UCLA before heading back to Colorado. I was invited by the head of a women's infertility support group, and the audience was mainly women with histories of infertility struggles and their partners. My presentation was very well received and to this day (since 2007) we still occasionally hear from someone who attended or a friend or loved one who has been referred to me.

This is what is meant by following your dharma—everything falls into place, you meet the right people at the right time; you are in harmony with the Universe. This is how the right clients are drawn to me: they are in harmony with their dharma, and they are at the place where they are ready to move to the next level. On a subconscious level they recognize that the sessions they do with me are what they need to align their energies with the energies of their babies. They know that subconsciously before I ever tell them. That's why they know they resonate with me.

We don't necessarily make the conscious choice to follow our life paths, but we do follow them to some extent. The Universe has ways of getting our attention, as I always tell my kids: the Universe will throw a rock in your path a few times; if you don't listen, eventually it will drop a boulder on you. You don't want the boulder. (My oldest son, an Indigo, totaled his car, then said he understood what I meant by a boulder!) For me, the weight loss program was a rock in my path, a distraction. Things went pretty well with it except I became progressively more and more drained. That's where the light bulb goes on (hopefully).

In harmony with my book, and with helping my clients bring their babies into the world, I carried on with working in my office, and with teaching my methods in various parts of the world. In 2008, as part of an awesome independent project, I was able to get my entire program accepted and recognized by the university where I was continuing my studies. I soon began accepting clients by phone—and then by Skype—as recognition of my work spanned the globe and not enough Certified HypnoFertility® therapists were accessible.

It's been at least three years since this book began churning in my mind, and a year since I finally committed to carrying a journal with me everywhere and entering every thought or word that had something to do with this topic. I came to recognize my pattern occurring; as I said, the Universe has its own way of working with me. I dissolved all association with an organization I discovered to be seriously lacking in integrity. I held a trainer training with a longtime friend and mentor of mine, Art Leidecker, aboard a Caribbean cruise ship. Art and I actually did several projects together with the HypnoFertility Foundation, a (non-profit) corporation I began in 2007 and which he and I revamped and partnered in from 2009 - 2012. I appeared on a show called *The Balancing Act* on Lifetime Television.

And I took on a weight loss counseling opportunity! I had to do it, I had wanted to do it years earlier, and even though I had all these other things going on, I told myself it would be a change of scenery, that it would be fun, that I could fit it in (in what Universe?). I had this strong intuitive drive to do it (though it certainly didn't make any logical sense), and it came together with ridiculous ease. I got to be a weight loss counselor for about the blink of an eye: the Universe just wanted to remind me of my life purpose, no doubt, and showered me with so many more fertility related projects I was in danger of drowning. Not to mention the personalities I'd encountered with many weight loss clients in the past still held precedence in the present.

My husband stood by quietly as what may have looked—to the ordinary eye at least—like a slight shift in everyday lifestyle unfolded as a spiritual leap. My husband, our office assistants, Molly and Martie, and I knew exactly, on one level or another, what was taking place. Martie even commented on the immediate energy shift. I laughed as I realized that the Universe had used the same reminder as before: weight loss. Are you listening, Lynsi? Write the book or we're sending the boulder!

The parallel reinforced my inner knowing: not only is my life purpose to connect spirit babies with their energetically aligned parents, I am the *Spirit Baby Whisperer*. This is my dharma—all roads lead here for me. It's not that I doubt it— I've been on board and paying attention all along—I just can't help but view it all from a humble standpoint, and am continually awed by the direction and loving reinforcement of the Universe, the Creator, of Source. The events leading up to this absolute declaration were to show me, yet again, my calling; the infinity symbol expressed: a Universal dedication to me, my dedication to the spirit babies.

Chapter 11

THE BALANCE OF INTENTION AND SURRENDER

*"If you have built castles in the air,
your work need not be lost; that is where they should be.
Now put foundations under them."*

—*Henry David Thoreau*

The balance of intention and surrender is the statement created by a client of mine who is both an attorney and a yoga instructor. I have always said that you "can't left brain a baby" and I still do. To me, the left brain represents science and medicine; the characteristics of logic, reason, decision making, and organization are traditionally attributed to it. If all you needed was science to conceive, the numbers would be much higher for IVF. With the technology we have currently we can retrieve the healthiest eggs, ensure fertilization, conduct genetic testing on the embryos, support the uterine lining to enhance implantation, etc. However, science alone does not produce success rates nearly as high as one would expect. With such capabilities, one might think that success rates in the 90% range would be more than likely.

This is where the right brain comes in. Creativity, imagination, emotion and such are attributed to the right brain. Creating a baby. Creation. It makes sense to enlist the skills of the right brain. And that's where the balance comes in. We must intend what we want to happen: I intend to have a baby. Then we must let go, we must surrender. When you mail a letter, you only mail it once. You don't keep fishing it out of the mailbox and putting it back in. It's done!

When you started on your fertility journey you intended to have a baby. You might have thought it would be much easier, or that it would have taken much less time. You might not have expected to need medical intervention or acupuncture or hypnosis. You did set the intention once, in some way at least, but now that you're here hypnosis can help you to subconsciously set the intention, create a healing state of balance, and effectively surrender (let go and let God).

We reinforce this mind state, release subconscious fears or blocks, and continually compound the hypnotic process with each session. I cannot address everything that needs attention in one session—there is simply too much—however I do begin by laying a powerful foundation and we build on it each week. Hypnosis is considered rapid change therapy though it still takes some time. Compared to acupuncture at twice per week for a year or more, or traditional therapy which is often once per week for several years, three months of hypnosis to conceive a baby is quite remarkable.

Even though we begin with the surrender piece, it often takes my clients time to be able to express it. They can intellectualize it but it's much harder for them to actually do it. Every client I have ever worked with has been a so-called and/or self-proclaimed Type-A personality. Each one has described herself in any or all of these terms: perfectionist, control freak, over-achiever, black-and-white thinker, workaholic, etc. I love Type-As, I am one; I totally get where the Type-A personality is coming from.

A quick word of clarification here: Type-A personality studies began in the 1950s and holes in the theory have been discovered over the years. The Type-A/Type-B personality designation is still recognized by the psychology field; it is quite prominent in pop psychology. The latter is more what we are speaking about here: this generalized interpretation of Type-A personalities as intense, stressed out, over-achieving, impatient, rigid, highly organized, perfectionistic, and workaholic; and Type-B personalities as easygoing, laid back, carefree, disorganized, flighty, non-driven, and even "starving-artist" is what those in our society tend to think of when we self-diagnose with these and other such labels. There is something to these designations as we know them, and I have great respect for the Type-A personality—they get things done. Type-As should not be converted into Type-Bs, nor should it be the other way around. Type-As just need to be in balance—that is to say, no throbbing neck veins or steam spewing from the ears!

Yes, Type-A personalities know how to "do." In bringing in the right brain attributes, in switching on the parasympathetic nervous system, in creating and maintaining the balance of mind, body, and spirit we are learning how to "be." You cannot *do being*. You can only *be*. This takes a bit of practice for my clients who are simply used to the fast paced, self-motivated style that permits corporate mergers or takeovers, financial acquisitions, catapulting to the top of the corporate ladder, pursuing a PhD while working a fulltime job, etc. I know you can *do* all of that, I know you can. But now it's time to *be*.

The Latin verb esse means "to be" says Dr. Marion Woodman. In discovering our own *being* she points out we are also discovering our essence (1985). This task is quite monumental when you consider that we have spent virtually our entire lives *doing*; and we must acknowledge that *doing* has become, in effect, an escape from *being*. *Being*, according to Woodman, is experienced as nothingness (1985).

Receptivity is crucial because you desire to receive your baby. Receptivity is the opposite of forcing, of doing, of pushing. As a woman your reproductive system is receptive to a man, you receive his sperm into your body. Lesbian women also receive sperm, perhaps not in a so-called traditional way, but they must receive it nonetheless. Your uterus receives an embryo, regardless of how that happens.

A receptive womb can envelop that tiny baby, nurture and nourish, and protect the baby until it's ready to enter the physical world. It's not that you have to give up everything, but a balance needs to occur, you must recognize the difference between what you can do (exercise, hypnosis, take medications, make/go to appointments, etc.) and what you must let go of (trying to force your ovaries to give you an egg the way you want it, telling God/dess what you want and when and how, spending countless hours scouring the internet to find something you want to hear and encountering a zillion things you didn't want to know).

Hypnosis gives you comfort and permission to stop trying. Try implies failure to the subconscious mind; trying (or doing) too hard often results in the complete opposite of what we desire. Tapping into the power of the subconscious mind removes the illusion of control, effectively supporting the surrender process and your ability to just be, to allow, to receive. I can see the surrender process. What I see is what connects between the head and the heart—one day it is just there and I know the baby is on its way. There is an energy, a "surrender-energy" if you will, that emanates from my clients' presence, voice, body language and overall vibration. It is apparent that the shift has occurred and she is now in proper alignment with her baby. I don't say anything; I just wait for the call.

Chapter 12

THE SACRED AND THE SUBCONSCIOUS

"I am a little pencil in the hand of a writing God who is sending a love letter to the world."

—*Mother Teresa*

As an author I view writing as a sacred duty. To be able to write is a gift; I know that I was given this gift as a part of my divine purpose and so I honor the process even more. A book can reach vast numbers of people. With the internet, anyone in the world can have access to the information I am setting forth here. I believe that books have an energy, a power of their own. I keep my spiritual books together on a bookshelf near my bed. I also have some of them on another bookshelf in my office. I feel I am absorbing their words, their ideals, and their energy while I work at my desk, while I meditate or read on my bed, virtually anytime I am near them.

I have a butsudan that contains my Gohonzon—a Buddhist scroll of devotion—on the top shelf of an antique bookcase. Below, the remaining shelves contain my various copies of spiritual writings including the *Bhagavad Gita*, the *Upanishads*, the *Dhammapada*, the *Tao Te Ching*, the *Bible*, and works of spiritual teachers like Ram Dass, Deepak Chopra, Eknath Easwaran, Wayne Dyer and Paramahansa Yogananda.

This is an energy center and simply being in its presence or sitting on the floor in front of it gives me great peace. I encourage my clients to set up such an area, even if it is one small space on the corner of a desk or table that contains one or two spiritual books or items. There is an intention in the action that speaks directly to the subconscious mind, and the subconscious mind is continuously impacted by the display whether you are thinking about it or not.

I believe we absorb energy from books, particularly spiritual or healing ones. Books; items such as a Buddha statue; rosary; candles depicting Jesus, Mary, guardian angels, the Divine Mother; plants; chimes or bells and other such things have a healing impact upon our energies. Healing music has a similar effect. My office is filled with soothing expressions of such healing energy: goddesses, fairies, angels, candles, and pictures; some given to me by appreciative clients and with the intention that they pass on their good fortune to others, some made for me by a dear Shaman friend, and some I acquired myself.

The energy in my office is incomparable. Clients immediately feel right at home when they enter. I have a burgundy colored beanbag chair—the metaphorical uterus—and my office has been nicknamed the womb room. Students at our training facility will often sneak away to relax in my office and, as they say, absorb the "good vibes." Our office assistant, Martie, enjoys meditating there. This is the energy of intention; this is the energy of surrender. When we allow ourselves to be open, to be receptive, we are able to benefit from such simple things. This energy transfers to my Skype and phone clients—I am the conductor.

I have been approached by women at lectures I've given, and they've told me the same thing about *It's Conceivable!* They feel they have absorbed the energy and that it has had a powerful effect on them. One woman was thrilled to tell me that she ordered my book and was pregnant before she'd finished reading it. This was after years of infertility and failed IVFs. Another, from out of state, called the office not long after receiving *It's Conceivable!* in the mail. She made an appointment with me and called back the next day to announce that she was pregnant. The ladies in our office get a kick out of some of the e-mails and calls we get.

One woman who was in a class my husband was teaching spoke to me of her infertility for a few minutes during a break while I happened to be there. Later I learned that she had bought my book with the intention of booking fertility sessions with me. When she came into my office she was about eight weeks pregnant. She got pregnant before she ever had time to book a session with me and so was coming in to do pregnancy work instead. She said she loved *It's Conceivable!* and had stayed up most of the night reading it the first time though she'd only intended to take in a chapter or two.

This was something she said she hadn't done since *Harry Potter* and I laughingly thanked her for the compliment, never having expected my little fertility book to be compared to bestselling fiction, let alone that of *Harry Potter* caliber. My client said she read *It's Conceivable!* four times, that she really connected with it, and that it had been really helpful to her. She said that it "read like literature" and—coming from someone with an English degree from Oxford—how could I not be pleased?

The feedback from readers, clients, and other therapists is a powerful reinforcement of the sacredness of the word, the all-pervading energy of books, the significance of quill to parchment. The power of intention radiates from certain writings and it is virtually palpable. What part of the brain is activated when we read spiritual or healing books? I would suggest perhaps that it has something to do with balance—the balance of intention and surrender; the shift into receptivity.

Chapter 13

THE FERTILITY VORTEX

"Manifestation is not magic. It is a process of working with natural principles and laws in order to translate energy from one level of reality to another."

—David Spangler

Long before I ever moved to Colorado I had heard that it was an energy mecca. The Rocky Mountains are filled with quartz crystal which amplifies energy, frequency, vibration. I have lived here for thirteen years now, but it didn't take long once I initially arrived for me to see and sense the effects of the majestic mountains. I wondered if I was actually living on or in a vortex, and I now know this to be true. What I mean by vortex, in this case, is spiraling spiritual energy. The energy flow exists in multiple dimensions, and interacts with an individual's spiritual gifts, chakras, and healing attributes.

It is no accident that two of the top fertility clinics in the world are located here in Colorado. The spirit baby work that I do is my life purpose and I know that the Universe arranged for me to end up here too. I created HypnoFertility® here. Shelley Torgrove, herbalist, healer, and proprietor of Artemesia & Rue, is a friend and colleague of mine who also completed my training. Shelley is an awesome woman who is essentially single-handedly responsible for bringing a very powerful fertility technique to the United States from Belize: Maya Abdominal Massage. Again, I believe this is due to the vortex.

Our area here is attracting those in need of fertility assistance through amplification of healing energy. This has influenced the healers too; we have aligned with the vortex energy, and simply accepted and integrated our natural gifts as the Universe guides our journeys. Combining the Divine Feminine and the vortex energy illuminates the power of intention, leading to the mind, body, and spirit balance that precedes receptivity—the balance of intention and surrender necessary for conception. Those of us who are properly aligned with the energy are able to transmit it. This energy is tangible in my office, but it also transmits through my Skype and phone sessions and accompanies me when I travel to teach. I don't have to do anything to cause this as it is simply the way it works; just the natural order of being.

Countless people have commented on my office over the years. With the vortex connection this time I will reiterate briefly. People often joke during school breaks that students have disappeared into the vortex (my office). Upon entering you are enveloped in soothing, healing energy similar to what you might notice walking into a church or labyrinth or out in nature. I have ordained my office carefully with specifically chosen items—powerful vortex conduits—intricately carved angel wings; various fertility Goddesses; sculpted turtles representing the Earth and fertility; and candles of Gabriel, Guadalupe, and rose. Many of these items were given to me as gifts—not just for me but to blend with the energy, to be shared with all client/baby matches occurring in and through my office. Again, that includes my distance clients: phone and Skype.

Listen

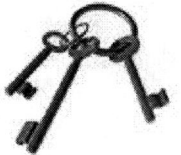

Chapter 14

THERE ARE TOO MANY PEOPLE ON THIS PLANET

*"There is a stubbornness about me that never can bear
to be frightened at the will of others.
My courage always rises at every attempt to intimidate me."*

—*Jane Austen*

Early on, as it became known that I am both a therapist and a teacher who helps women get pregnant, and/or trains others in my HypnoFertility® methods, some people—even other therapists—scorned what I was doing because "there are already too many people on this planet/we don't need more babies/the planet is overpopulated." Many of my clients have encountered the same type of attitude, be it from friends, family, or co-workers, or from healthcare providers. I think it is a statement of ignorance, and I have said so many times.

It is no one's place to pass judgment on yours or anyone's desire to have children. Tactless statements to the effect of "maybe it's not God's plan/you can just adopt/there are too many people on this planet" do not come from a place of knowing; they come from ego. They come from the fear-based, controlling, left brain aspect of human expression; they are nothing more than opinion. We are all entitled to our own opinions, though I often wish people would actually look up the meaning of the word. An opinion, by its very nature, cannot be wrong; but it is also not fact or truth—it is a sentiment, a belief, a conviction.

There are certain types of people who will challenge your opinions, who don't accept the idea that everyone can have one. Someone's opinion may not match the facts; presented as fact their reasoning may well be wrong, but not in the form of an opinion. This is why I recommend keeping your fertility journey to yourself. Insensitive remarks in this respect don't bother me; however, when you are emotionally vulnerable, overwhelmed, and frightened—when it is your personal reality at stake—such foolish statements can pierce to your core.

Interestingly, people with children of their own have made similar statements to me and to my clients. In these cases I can only imagine what kind of shadow lurks behind the mask they show to the world. What kinds of wounds lie unraveled in their psyches, unattended, deep and dark? Emotionally unbuttoned, yet unaware, these people spew sweet poison from their lips; sugar coated counsel with a venomous sting. This is why you must clear your energy, and why you must learn to shield. Both of these are automatic inclusions in my private client sessions, they don't take long but have powerful effects. The *Cancel Technique*, as outlined in *It's Conceivable!*, is helpful here too.

It is important to guard against malicious, opinionated, ignorant, or simply unaware remarks regarding your fertility. It is essential to have techniques you can use to counter them if you must, but remember that you don't owe explanations to anyone—including your own parents. You must discern what is in the best interest of your baby. Of you, your partner, and your baby. If you don't have a partner—particularly if you don't have a partner because you won't have that intimate type of support available to you—then you must focus on your baby and you. This starts pre-conception but it continues throughout pregnancy, birth, and beyond.

I tell my clients to utilize their team. Their team is me, their Maya massage practitioner, their acupuncturist, or massage therapist, or chiropractor, etc. Whomever they are working with comprises the client's team. This is where you are safe, and this is where you get recharged. If clients have supportive friends or family, they can include them in their team at their discretion. I ask them to discern carefully.

There is comfort in feeling yourself surrounded in loving, supportive, spiritual energy that helps maintain the balance of mind, body, and spirit we are working on right from the first session. From this space you emit the energy frequency that is in harmony with your baby's, to create the alignment necessary for your baby to transition from the spiritual world into the physical one. All of this reinforces the hypnosis aspect of the *Spirit Baby Whisperer* process: keeping the subconscious mind on task and, therefore, all systems and organs in effective function.

According to Harvard-trained neuroanatomist Jill Bolte Taylor (2006) our right brain is the hemisphere that perceives the big picture. It recognizes that virtually everything: everything around us, everything about us, everything among and within us is comprised of particles of energy that are woven together into a universal tapestry. With everything connected we find an intimate relationship between the atomic space that is around us and within us no matter where we are. From an energetic standpoint, says Taylor, if we think about someone, send good vibrations his or her way, hold someone in the light, or pray for an individual, then we are consciously sending our own energy to that person with a healing intention (2006). If we meditate upon a person or lay our hands upon someone's wound, then we are directing the energy of our beings purposefully to help someone to heal.

Exactly how the arts of Reiki, hypnosis, and prayer (to mention only a few) work remain to this day medical mysteries to some extent. In her brilliant book *My Stroke of Insight* Dr. Taylor (2006) explains that this is basically because our left brains and science have simply not yet caught up with what we recognize to be true about the way our right hemisphere functions. She does believe, however, that our right minds are "perfectly clear about how they intuitively perceive and interpret energy dynamics" (Taylor, 2006, p. 169).

To create energetic balance, Dr. Taylor recommends listening to a verbal meditation/hypnosis recording that guides you into an emotionally and even physiologically impressed thought pattern that will shift your mind away from unwanted loops (2006). This is precisely what is happening with the HF recordings I have you work with and why it is essential to support your brain—and your mind, body, and spirit—consistently in this manner. Prayer is another method of using our minds to deliberately replace unwanted, negative thought patterns with a chosen set of positive, healing thought patterns. This is simply one more way to consciously direct one's mind away from the incessant verbal repetition hamster wheel and into a more peaceful place.

If they're not going through it, people don't know what you are experiencing and they may ask inappropriate questions. I consider infertility to be a catastrophic condition (such as cancer). As a hypnotherapist, I don't use the word infertility unless it is in initially identifying the issue. I don't exactly call it a "catastrophic" issue because, again, that is not correct hypnotic "speak." Words that cause a strong mental reaction, that easily form a picture, that stir the emotions, in hypnosis are called painted words. "He crunched his knee," or "she shattered her hand" are just a couple of examples—you probably cringed when you read each one. Like a painting, the effect is instantaneous upon the forefront of your mind.

It is essential, however, that my clients receive the kindness afforded to those with cancer and other such serious conditions. I spent several years early on in my practice working with a noteworthy friend and mentor, Dr. C. Scot Giles, who specializes in oncology hypnosis. It is because I had the foresight to accept this extraordinary opportunity that I can see this unrecognized parallel; I appreciate the emotional devastation that often accompanies fertility issues, but often others do not. When someone discloses that they have cancer, people will usually offer sympathy, or perhaps ask if there is anything they can do. When women disclose that they have infertility, they are usually met with less than sensitive remarks: a sweeping gesture of the arm and a "que sera, sera" type of statement, "you can just adopt, lots of kids need homes," or a kind of "oh well."

Having endured this type of experience countless times by the time they get to me, my clients are in dire need of support and empathy. And they also need tools: techniques to free them from vulnerability, to give them hope, to help them rally their strengths, and, in effect, to press the reset button. In essence, the fertility formula: rapid, effective, personal; because, in so many cases, time is running out.

Chapter 15

MY PEOPLE ARE COMING

"I think I was born strong-willed. That's not the kind of thing you can learn. The advantage is, you stick to what you believe in and rarely get pushed out of what you want to do."

—Joan Jett

I recall being little, maybe three-years-old, and sitting on the thick, deep, concrete steps that led to the front door of my childhood home. My dad came out at some point and asked what I was doing. I told him I was waiting for my real people to come get me. He laughed. I didn't find it funny—only annoying that he should laugh, should not take me seriously. I turned away from him, wedged my elbows against my knees, dropped my chin into my hands, and proceeded to wait. They didn't come.

I was sure my people were going to come and get me—if there was one thing I knew for certain it was that I didn't belong in that house, or with that family. I was sensitive, right from the get-go. I was creative, imaginative, had a very high IQ. I entered the world a vegetarian and in the Southern Ontario area of Canada in the late sixties that did not go over well. I was an introvert, and didn't want to play with anybody. I preferred adult conversation when I could get it. I started kindergarten at age three, and my teacher wrote home in my report card that I "tolerated" the other children.

At one point I saw the Bugs Bunny cartoon with "Yob." A couple go to the hospital to have a baby. The husband falls asleep while his wife is in the delivery room and he dreams that his baby (Yob, which is boy spelled backward) was switched with an alien. A light bulb went on and I was certain that that must have been what had happened to me, except that in my case it was not a dream. My parents informed me that this was impossible, that it just wasn't reality. It seemed to me that I saw "reality" a lot differently than most people I spent my childhood with.

I believe we choose our parents, and that we have lessons to learn that help us carry out our life purposes. I always say that if you want to get tough, try growing up a vegetarian child in a working class Toronto west end suburb during the early seventies. I must have really wanted to get tough, because I set myself up for a heck of an ordeal with that choice. I've often wondered if I'm a reincarnated Buddha. Whatever the case, I came through to this world with a very different view than most people I encountered.

The kids I went to school with taunted me for not eating hotdogs. If anything should have turned me—made me conform—it should have been that. They were quite cruel about it. Parents were worse in a sense. They said I couldn't come over to their houses because I "didn't eat anything." That wasn't actually true, I ate—just not meat. I think they thought I would die on them as from what I could see people who didn't eat meat starved to death quite rapidly and consistently. My parents forced me to eat it, and I have often remarked that if you had a time machine and went back to any day of my childhood you would find me sitting at the kitchen table long after suppertime in front of a hunk of meat. Thank God for 1978 when we got a dog!

I got so that when I had to eat meat I would swallow it whole. I don't know how good that was for my digestive system but it sure beat biting down on those awful hard things that make a popping sound in your mouth. I never cracked—

no matter how much I was yelled at, threatened or ridiculed—and once I was on my own I stopped eating all of it. I'm still alive, and I have to wonder if my meat resistance journey was so that I could relate to these new and even more sensitive babies. And I am tough—didn't give into peer pressure even when I was a tiny girl. I believed in myself then and I do now; this is how I am able to hold the space for my clients. I don't judge any situation; I simply help to process it, if that's what needs to happen.

In *The Children of Now* Losey (2007) reports that because these special children are so advanced intellectually, spiritually, and emotionally they suffer from a great sense of not belonging. Because they come from a frame of reference that is quite foreign to most people in this world, many of these brilliant children remain unheard, invalidated, and unacknowledged. This happened a great deal more with the Indigos of my generation; this is why certain babies—the babies I work with—are choosing parents who will see to it that their needs are met in a way that will support their purpose. If your child desires to be a vegetarian, for example, you will not resist. If your child is a loner she will be supported, if your child is interested in meditation or yoga you will not find it odd. Also, these special little beings want education so they need parents who will encourage them, and make sure they get it.

Chapter 16

THE POWER OF THE PAST

"The soul always knows what to do to heal itself.
The challenge is to silence the mind."

—*Caroline Myss*

A popular reason that people come to see hypnotherapists is for a Past Life Regression (PLR). The idea, here, is to be regressed back in time to a time that your subconscious mind deems necessary for your healing or understanding (or both). With a hypnotic PLR you actually do the time travel, and you actually have the experience. Some people have had psychic Past Life Regressions in which the psychic reads the lifetimes out of your energy and tells you what they are. Personally, I don't think those are as much fun since you don't get to participate. For fertility purposes I will occasionally do a PLR, usually around the mid to latter part of a client's session series.

It is possible that a subconscious block is coming from a past life. If you were a washer woman with twelve children and not enough food, for example, you might have made a pact with yourself not to have children in your next life. Whether or not you actually said or meant next life, a vehement intention to that effect is enough to impact your subconscious mind. Even if you do not believe in past lives (they can be explained as tapping into the collective unconscious, or metaphor, or soul memories, etc.) a PLR can be a very powerful mechanism in releasing subconscious blocks.

Transformational Replay is present life regression, or regression for short (Also sometimes called age regression). My husband, Drake, has written a fabulous book on the subject entitled *The Power of the Past* (the inspiration for this chapter title). Drake selected an accurate title for his book in that hypnotic regression can facilitate powerful healing in a relatively short time. There are other ways to release subconscious blocks and these can be done in the office, by phone, or by Skype. Because of the interactive process necessary for true regression I prefer to do regression of any kind in the office.

I rarely use regressions with HF. I consider them the heavy artillery—to be used if absolutely necessary. But I almost never need them. Both my husband and I feel that clients get more benefit from the deep hypnosis methods we utilize and this is what we teach our hypnotherapy students. Regression has to be done from a lighter state of hypnosis and for best results clients should have at least four sessions before it is used. I can tell if regression is necessary, and I will mention it if I think it pertinent. I also have an excellent protocol so that my distance clients may benefit from regression should they and I believe it necessary.

I mention both regression and PLR here because they are certainly hypnotic buzz words and you may well have heard them before. I also detail a regression in *It's Conceivable!* and occasionally mention regression in this book as well. It was what we call a Life Purpose Regression that I experienced when I met the little spirit babies several years ago. All forms of regression can be quite awesome—under the right circumstances. I believe it's important to know what they are, and also to know that very few of the babies whose births I have helped to facilitate had mothers who needed regression.

Hypnosis is unsurpassed at releasing subconscious blocks and I do so with all my clients. There are many effective techniques that do this work more quickly and easily than regression. I am not against regression, I just know that if a person gets her mind set on something like that and it is not necessary or it is done prematurely it can cause setbacks that she does not want. I desire to explain the above processes to you for the purpose of understanding, and so that you will know that there are so many options with HypnoFertility®. I also know that women dealing with infertility tend to scour the internet looking, reading, researching; stirring up their stress levels to preposterous heights in the name of self-education.

Messages from the Masters (Weiss, 2000) points out that letting go of fear, anger, and other negative emotions is essential to both good physical health and spiritual well-being. According to Weiss (2000), it is now widely recognized that mental stress (including negative emotions such as fear, anger, chronic anxiety, and depression) is one of the prime causes of illness and death in the entire world. Because our bodies are intimately linked to our minds, it makes perfect sense that our moods and emotions are easily translated into physical symptoms—unexplained infertility is just one example. "Love can heal; stress can kill" (Weiss, 2000).

Significantly considered to be the top general medical journal in the United States the *New England Journal of Medicine* published a major article in January of 1998 (as cited in Weiss, 2000). This impressive piece addressed specifically the multi-system damage that chronic stress can and does impose upon the human body. A complex system of hormones and other chemicals are released into the body in response to mental stress, and if these hormones are not rapidly inactivated—often because the stress persists and the body continues to produce these chemicals—organs in our bodies become exposed to dire consequences. As we know, stress causes changes in heart rate, blood pressure; it impacts organs and systems throughout the body. Stress can be devastating; stress must be addressed.

The goal of this work is to help you achieve and maintain balance of mind, body, and spirit. The HF program is holistic and carefully designed to address your every need— and those of your baby(s). Working together with your therapist and trusting the process is your most direct route to the success you desire. Remember to limit your time on the internet and in any chat rooms or message boards so that you are able to maintain your overall balance.

Chapter 11

THE EXIT AND THE ENTRANCE

"Love is something eternal;
the aspect may change, but not the essence."

—*Vincent Van Gogh*

I find that one of the easiest ways to explain the presence of spirit babies is to compare it to what happens in hospice. Anyone who has worked in or had a family member or friend in hospice knows that there is a certain energy present. As death draws near, the person begins to have conversations with loved ones who have passed on, and often they will report that their mother or older brother or spouse (or other loved one) who passed on before them has come to meet them. Some days their eyes will light up as they stare into what appears to be space; sometimes they'll gaze dreamily for hours. There is a sense of contentment at these times, of peace, and of trust.

Anyone I have ever met who has been closely involved in hospice care—from medical professionals to laypersons—has told me that it changed them, that they no longer fear death, and that the spiritual energy they've experienced is palpable. They come to recognize hospice as just an exit from the physical realm. Similarly, a client of mine has a sister who is a neurosurgeon in Ireland. This brilliant doctor honors both her late mother and her Irish Catholic heritage each time a patient dies by opening a window. To let the spirit out, she was taught.

Well, not only do spirits leave this world, but they also enter it. I liken my work to a sort of "reverse hospice" where I can feel the energy as the babies prepare to enter this world. Their mothers sense them too or have dreams about them. The babies, like sparkly little bubbles, float in and around their mothers' auras. They consider themselves alive and present in their parents' lives; the parents, in most cases, simply don't know or understand that.

As I explain to my clients, you already are a mother to your spirit baby; it's just a matter of time until your baby comes through to the physical world. That's what things like timed intercourse or Clomid or IUI, etc. are for—to help you create a body for your baby. Your baby is already here. My HypnoFertility® process provides you the assistance to align the energies so that your spirit baby can shift to a soon-to-be newborn baby.

Chapter 18

THE NECESSARY MINDSET

"Science without religion is lame, religion without science is blind."

—*Einstein*

Many of my clients consider themselves spiritual rather than religious but I have found that even those of a more traditional Christian faith (or Jewish, or atheist, etc.) accept and appreciate Buddhist principles. Though it is characterized as an Eastern religion, I tend to view Buddhism as more of a philosophy. Buddhism radiates such gentleness; it is a splendid example of some of the very faculties we are addressing here: surrender, detachment, mindfulness, meditation.

Surrender is basically something you cannot do—it is a state of *being* you must cultivate just as we discussed earlier. The work that you do to create your own healing—the tools you use to *let go and let God* so to speak—facilitate surrender. You become one with surrender as you follow your heart, your path, and your intuition; as you honor the 3 keys: meditate, listen, and trust. You are right, in some ways surrender is a paradox (I will address this further in the following chapter).

However, it is also a quest that you must master—your baby is waiting.

Detachment, from a Buddhist standpoint, is basically the separation from all that there is in the world. It's not that you can't have what you want, but that you cultivate a "take-it-or-leave-it" attitude. In seeing the goods of the world as less than permanent, less enticing than we might once have thought, we find ourselves detached from pains as well as pleasures. Through this practice we are able to take the sting out of life's injustices and trust that all will unfold as necessary (my baby is coming in just the right time and in just the right way). Detachment dovetails seamlessly with the balance of mind, body, and spirit.

Mindfulness, according to Buddhist monk Thich Nhat Hahn, is the recognition of what is *there* be it negative or positive (2001); to embrace it and get in touch with it. We must recognize that our goal is not to fight—for example taking care of the emotion of anger should it arise, says Hahn. For the purpose of realizing that which we have not acknowledged before, it is important to look deeply within. The practice of mindful breathing and mindful walking generates mindfulness energy. The energy of mindfulness contains the energy of concentration and the energy of insight (Hahn, 2001).

Meditation activates the peripheral nervous system (PNS) through multiple pathways (Hanson, 2009). Through stimulating the PNS as well as other parts of the nervous system attention is withdrawn from stressful matters while awareness is brought to the body. Stimulation of the PNS and other parts of the nervous system through regular meditation affects the brain in numerous ways including: increasing gray matter in the insula (Hölzel et al., 2008 as cited in Hanson, 2009), hippocampus (Hölzel et al., 2008; Luders et al., 2009 as cited in Hanson, 2009), and prefrontal cortex (Lazar, 2005; Luders et al., 2009 as cited in Hanson, 2009).

According to Davidson (2004 as cited in Hanson, 2009) activation of the left frontal regions of the brain are increased during meditation which lifts mood. Stress-related cortisol is released (Tang et al., 2007 as cited in Hanson 2009) and the immune system is strengthened (Davidson et al., 2003; Tang et al., 2007 as cited in Hanson, 2009). Meditation is shown to help a wide variety of issues including—but not limited to—cardiovascular disease, asthma, type II diabetes, PMS, and chronic pain (Walsh and Shapiro, 2006 as cited in Hanson, 2009).

Brain research conducted by Drs. Andrew Newberg and the late Eugene D'Aquili earlier this decade have helped Dr. Jill Bolte Taylor—herself a brain scientist—to understand what was happening in her brain exactly. With the aid of SPECT technology (single photon emission computed tomography) these scientists were able to identify the neuroanatomy underlying our ability to have a religious or spiritual (mystical) experience (2006). Their goal was to understand which regions of the brain were involved in our ability to undergo a shift in consciousness—in other words to go away from being an individual to feeling that we are at *one* with the universe (God, Nirvana, euphoria).

Taylor, in her book *My Stroke of Insight* (2006) explains some impressive research in which Tibetan meditators and Franciscan nuns were asked to meditate or pray inside the SPECT machine. Monks and nuns alike were instructed to tug on a piece of cotton twine as soon as they reached their meditative climax or felt united with God. These significant experiments identified shifts in neurological activity in regions in the brain that were very specific. First, they found that there was a decrease in the activity of the language centers of the left hemisphere that resulted in a silencing of their brain chatter. Also, there was a decrease in activity in the orientation association area, found in the posterior parietal gyrus of the left hemisphere. According to scientists, this region of our left brain helps us to identify our personal physical boundaries; this, to me, reinforces the need to balance the brain hemispheres and emphasizes the essential balance of mind, body, and spirit (Why God Won't Go Away 2001, as cited in Taylor, 2006).

Herbert Benson, MD, the Harvard Cardiologist whose book *The Relaxation Response* (1975) brought mind/body healing to the forefront of the minds of the general public, says that as a society in general we tend to give traditional medicine far too much power over ourselves. He concurs with the Buddhist standpoint that we are putting too much focus on external techniques while all but ignoring our own inner techniques. Benson also prescribes balance using an analogy of a three-legged stool. He believes we need all three for optimal health: traditional medical care, alternative/complementary care, and self-care.

This is not to say that conventional medicine is unnecessary, or that any of us think so. I work in tandem with reproductive endocrinologists regularly, as do Mayan massage workers, acupuncturists, etc. As with anything, there are some people who are totally open and others who are completely closed. There are also a good many that are in the process of shifting perception because something has occurred in their lives that calls for them to take notice.

Benson is a pioneer in the mind/body medicine movement. He experimented with a technique he termed the relaxation response, based initially on transcendental meditation. At his mind/body institute in the Boston area, he has conducted a number of studies over several decades. His method was also cited in some of the research of his colleague, Dr. Alice Domar. Much of Dr. Domar's research is some of the best to support the success of hypnotherapy for infertility; Dr. Benson affirms in *The Relaxation Response* that the same effects are induced with both the relaxation response and hypnotherapy. The same physiological changes were also noted with autogenic training, Zen and yoga, and transcendental meditation.

My husband, Drake Eastburn, wrote a much needed book for contemporary hypnotism: *What is Hypnosis?* (2010). Not only does it quash misconceptions and mysteries about this phenomenal modality, his book literally ties it all together and precisely defines each word, each ideology, every meaning, every contention, virtually all of hypnotism and it's understudies. An incredible amount of research went into this book and with good reason. Because of Drake, contemporary hypnotism is becoming clearer and more concise than ever before. Dr. Benson states in his book that hypnosis in not well-understood, and many people have some serious misconceptions of the process. John Gruzilier of the Imperial College of Medicine in London has written a very perceptive paper on how hypnosis must not be defined; the Mayo Clinic (as cited in *It's Conceivable!*) also has some enlightening information on the subject on their website.

The *Buddhism of Nichiren Daishonin* (Causton, 1995) tells us that one of the fastest ways to change any personal problem is to work diligently toward the fundamental happiness of others. The idea, though it may sound paradoxical, is that in concerning yourself with the happiness of others, your life expands so that you are no longer dominated by an introspective and suffocating focus upon your own issues. Adding one drop of ink to a cup of water turns all the water blue; added to the ocean, the same drop of ink will disappear altogether. In other words, according to the wisdom of Nichiren Daishonin, (Causton, 1995), in gradually expanding your life by making efforts to assist others, you not only reduce your suffering, you simultaneously develop the strengths of wisdom, compassion, and courage, which in turn you apply to your own issues.

Central to the practice of Buddhism is the understanding that both happiness and suffering come from within. In shifting the fundamental attitude, suffering dissipates. Such is also true with hypnotherapy and thus the parallel in philosophies. Rather than trying to revamp Buddhism in its entirety (as I have seen others actually attempt), I prefer to draw from its wisdom and incorporate the pieces that resonate with my clients in ways that support their individual journeys.

An analogy of a lotus flower is expressed in *The Buddha in Daily Life* (Causton, 1995). Only because the lotus flower's roots are so deeply buried in the muck of the swamp is it able to bloom so exquisitely. That is to say that the "muck" we must trudge through in our ordinary lives—human desires, human problems—is the root of our desire to change, to blossom. Your fertility issues are a gift: they have led you to seek true healing and to commit to it; the fact that you have this book in your hands right now shows your dedication—your own lotus has already begun to sprout.

I have explained the necessary mindset for overcoming fertility, pregnancy, and birthing issues, and I reiterate it briefly here from a Buddhist and medical standpoint. Mind/body medicine is becoming increasingly popular in traditional Western medicine. My husband and I regularly receive medical referrals and maintain professional relationships with medical doctors, reproductive clinics, psychiatrists, staff from mental health facilities including Denver's Fort Logan, etc. Doctors and therapists at Kaiser Permanente (a very contained healthcare facility) refer patients to us (outside their network). Even so, many people do not realize that the most powerful medicine lies within them, that their very own attitudes and determination greatly impact their healing.

The key, here, is not to place all one's faith in healing in an outside force such as a medical facility because being told that something is incurable (old eggs) or virtually impossible (you have a less than 1% chance of conception—IVF or otherwise) by such an authority figure as a doctor can cause not only complete loss of hope, but loss of all chance of recovery as well. In such cases this type of diagnosis can hit hard—like a death sentence—knocking into your gut, your heart, and other areas, distressing your chakra energies, and taking firm hold within your subconscious mind.

What I have always conceded is this: hypnosis contains all of the above mentioned techniques; each can induce deep relaxation. The difference is that hypnosis is a heavy hitter—when relaxation is not enough we can help you to utilize the hypnotic process to remove fears or blocks from your subconscious mind. I could have disguised HypnoFertility® by calling it *Guided Fertility Relaxation* or *Creative Fertility* or something. I could have done what Jose Silva did in the 1970s which was to avoid the word hypnosis and call his technique *Silva Mind Control* (that's any less scary?!) which is now known as the *Silva Method*. I didn't because I know the healing power hypnosis has and I wanted to distinguish the process.

To explain a little more clearly, there are three major ways we approach infertility with hypnosis: one is that we utilize very deep trance (relaxation) to address the parasympathetic nervous system and/or stress. Secondly, we use visualization/imagery/analogy/meditation/metaphor and various suggestion methods (based on intake) for clearing and repatterning; resetting inherent abilities (such as intuition). The third method is what we in the hypnotism field refer to as interactive process: gestalt, parts therapy, regression to cause, PLR, Life Purpose Regression. As you can see we have awesome firepower when we tap into hypnotism as a whole. In so doing, we are able to access, activate, and adhere to the 3 keys: meditate, listen, trust.

For healing infertility or anything else we need a balance of mind, body, and spirit. We need our inside force (our minds, our spirits) to balance any outside force—when we have that anything is possible, miracles happen. My practice is full of miracles: natural (healthy) conceptions for women at 43, 44, 45, 46, 47, 48, and even 49 (supposedly impossible); women down to their "last chance" with nothing left but a single frozen 4-cell embryo giving birth to healthy babies . . . and those are just a few. Miracles are possible! Miracles are *abundant* through attainment of balance.

Chapter 19

THE TRUTH ABOUT SURRENDER

You must learn to be still in the midst of activity
and to be vibrantly alive in repose.

—*Indira Ghandi*

The meanings of surrender from what we've learned in the Western culture, and from what it means in the East must be compared and contrasted. From our social standpoint it basically means to give up or to give in; according to Merriam-Webster (2012): "to yield to the power, control, or possession of another upon compulsion or demand." We are taught to fight; we are encouraged to never give up no matter how bad things are. From a Western view we are in a perpetual warzone of control; always trying, always struggling to control. Surrender is virtually the end from this standpoint, and we resist with all our might.

Surrender in the Eastern traditions such as Buddhism, is an art or a concept that literally means to stop fighting. That is, says Dr. Amy Johnson (2012), to stop fighting yourself: the Universe, the natural flow of things, and to stop resisting your reality. For victims of control issues, perfectionist tendencies and overall Type-A characteristics, the Eastern application of surrender creates an energy much more resourceful than—what is actually an illusion of—control could ever be.

In other words, it's not about giving up, but about going forth from the energy of surrender; honoring the ebb and flow or *yin and yang* of your life path. As I have so often expressed to my clients, it's a matter of *being* rather than *doing*—that balance between intent and surrender that enables you to effectively *Let go and let God*. Or *give it to the Universe, release it to the Divine Mother, invite the angels to take it*; however you would like to term it.

In understanding surrender, we must also understand that when humans shift into a protective mode they will unavoidably restrict their growth behaviors. If you're trying to run away from a lion, then it is not such a great idea to expend energy on growth (Lipton, 2005). In order to survive—to just escape that lion—all of your energy must be summoned for your fight or flight response. The redistribution of energy reserves to fuel the protection response inevitably equals a curtailment of growth. Inhibiting growth processes is debilitating—growth is a process that both expends energy and is also required to produce it.

A sustained fight or flight response inhibits the creation of life-sustaining energy. The longer you stay in protection, the more your growth is compromised. We have 50 trillion cells of which not all must be in growth or protection mode at the same time, says Lipton (2005). The percentage of cells in a protective response depends on the severity of perceived threats. What Dr. Lipton says that is crucial to pay attention to is this: chronic inhibition of growth mechanisms poses severe compromises to your life, energy, vitality; just getting rid of stressors is not enough to heal in and of itself. Lipton (2005) tells us in no uncertain terms how essential it is to seek joyful, loving, peaceful activities, and to create lives as such, so that we not only live but are able to thrive, and to stimulate the growth process. In other words, to surrender.

Our physiology has not yet caught up to contemporary society. Our fight or flight response is designed to protect us from danger—imminent danger such as a wild animal that we must fight off or flee from quickly. For this reason our body mobilizes its energies: pulls blood and oxygen away from systems deemed inessential to survival—such as the reproductive system—and directs all stores toward raising high alert of the crucial-to-survival heart, lungs, eyes, arms and legs, and so forth. This mechanism creates a burst of energy, of enhanced bodily function, that is designed to save your life. The process is quite effective under such circumstances.

The problem we have is that though human beings have evolved some since ancient times, our recent catapult into sophisticated technology, into the so-called information age, has left our DNA in the dust. Our sympathetic nervous systems are running on a model that consists of wild animals; dangerous cliffs or caves; miles of walking, hunting, foraging for food; building and rebuilding camps or living quarters and the like. It is not tuned in to deal with heavy, emotional, on-going stressors like financial worries or infertility. Mortgage fears, for example, are there day by day, hanging over your head, causing the fight or flight response to turn on and stay on. Worries, invasive fertility procedures, high costs of medical treatments, uncertainty of outcome—the all-and-out fear that is constant and consistent during the infertility trek elicits the same response as the ongoing mortgage worries: a continual dousing of organs and systems by a flood of dangerous and damaging stressor hormones.

It doesn't have to be this way. There are ways to override the fight or flight response, to shift from the sympathetic nervous system to the parasympathetic. I use the analogy of a cat to explain this to my clients. Imagine a cat walking leisurely through a garden. He's fine, he's happy; it's just a normal day for the cat. Suddenly, a ferocious sounding dog comes running over from behind a house. His teeth are bared, his eyes are on our furry friend, and he is growling and snapping. Looking at the cat you see his hackles rise, his claws shoot out; he yowls and takes off, virtually flying up into a tall, out-of-dog-reach tree.

The dog looks longingly upward and barks awhile; eventually he either gets bored or someone shoos him away.

After a bit the cat scouts the area below, determines it is safe to come down, and descends the tree. A moment or so later you see that the cat is flopped in the grass licking his fur. All is right with the world. I joke with my clients that what we're missing as humans is that we don't lick our fur. We have a little chuckle and we nod that it is true.

The cat did not sit up in the tree and call a bunch of friends on his cell phone, telling his story over and over. He did not shift into a fearful negative thinking pattern about how dangerous the garden is and how he'll have to avoid it. He just laid down in the sunshine and licked his fur. That is how our physiology is designed to function: a quick mobilization of energies and a choice of fight or flee; once out of danger the parasympathetic nervous system kicks in and we are in rejuvenation mode.

Cats don't have mortgages, I know. The cat's lifestyle enables him to function in harmony with his nervous system. He doesn't have to make an effort to balance, but as humans, we do. The good news is that we can override or reset the fight or flight switch. It must be done on an ongoing basis; it must become a way of life. Daily hypnosis and/or meditation—even if for just a few minutes—balances, and reinforces balance, of the sympathetic and parasympathetic nervous systems.

Surrender to God is a requirement of every religion, to the extent that it is far too great a subject to be addressed here. There certainly is spiritual connection to the HF process (religious as well should you wish to include it), though preference makes no difference. Surrender, as I have explained it here, is a key component in your healthy conception. It's not always easy to surrender—though HF helps extensively with that—but once you've truly done it the shift in energy is astounding and virtually palpable to genuine Sensitives, Intuitives, lightworkers, and healers, alike.

Chapter 20

THE POWER OF WORDS

"Better than a thousand hollow words, is one word that brings peace."

—*Buddha*

Recently, a colleague of ours gave a talk at our office. I have been the president of the National Guild of Hypnotists Denver chapter meeting since January 2000. Over the past few years my husband and I have pretty much split that position due, mainly, to both our busy teaching schedules (and our inability to be in two places at once!). The meeting takes place the third Thursday evening of every month (ten or eleven months each year), and we invite speakers we hope will have a topic that is interesting, and even complementary, to the certified hypnotherapists who make up our membership.

Dr. Cody Horton is a stage hypnotist and also does a great deal of corporate work in and around the Denver area. Cody has taught classes for the Institute and she is always a popular guest speaker at the meetings. Her latest talk was about *Quantum Creating* and as she presented her topic my mind drifted off in that delicious hypnotic waking/dream state that enables me to pay attention while at the same time subconscious awareness takes the forefront.

I have been gathering information for inclusion in this book for quite some time. My subconscious (the most powerful goal-achieving agent on the planet) mind knows this and is constantly keeping on the lookout for tidbits of information my clients and readers need to have. (Just as I use unparalleled hypnotic techniques to connect my clients to their babies, so do I benefit from them as well.) This was the case here.

Cody was teaching about the power of words which is a topic always of interest to hypnotherapists (sales and marketing people also, by the way). It is particularly important what words are delivered to the subconscious mind and how. Drake and I always teach our certification students and advanced class students the importance of *painted words*. The subconscious mind responds to pictures, imagery, emotion (such as drama), metaphor, allegory, and story. This is crucial because painted words cause the action of the word to occur: relax, headache, breathe, pain. And/or these words hold a charge that causes us to instantaneously imagine and emotionally respond to them: the child was ripped from her loins (a grimace, shudder, verbal expression such as ouch).

Cody discussed how the word *but* negates the sentence before it while *because* is very powerful. When we hear someone say something that is followed by a *but*, we tend to respond negatively, possibly discounting their point or explanation completely, and that response impacts the subconscious mind more strongly than what they had initially started out to convey. *Because* tells us why. It gets our attention *because* our minds are conditioned to believe that things work if you can provide a *because*. *But* and *because* are not painted words, however they are important because used in therapeutic hypnosis, or used within self-hypnosis suggestion or affirmation, they can work for you or against you.

- Your baby is coming to you because you are creating balance.

- Your baby is coming to you but you must create balance.

- Don't worry about your infertility.

- Your fertility is rich and lush.

The first statement is a good hypnotic suggestion using *because* to reinforce the suggestion of creating balance. (For a hypnotherapist, there is actually more to it than even that; as a client, you see the example of what is explained above.) In the second statement the same positive statement is given as in the first example. This time, though, *but* discounts it: but you must create balance. You are creating and you must create two different things. The former is in present tense, the latter is in future tense. The subconscious mind recognizes only the present tense; there is no past or future tense in the subconscious mind. (Therefore, suggestions given in this manner are immediately discounted by the subconscious mind.)

The third sentence is a doozy from a hypnotic standpoint. *Don't* is not recognized by the subconscious mind. This is a hypnosis phenomenon called pharsing: *Don't* think of a pink elephant. What happens when you hear that? The pink elephant immediately pops into your mind because you have to think of it in order to *not* think of it.

Worry, as you now know, is a painted word. Your nervous system will readily respond to the idea/image/feeling of worry. Plus, by saying *don't worry* you are in effect instructing the person to *worry*. *Infertility* is a charged word and can act as a powerful reinforcement to whatever the issue might be—the subconscious knows whether we do or not. Don't worry about your infertility could produce a subconscious response of negative stressor hormones being directed to the ovaries, for example.

Your fertility is rich and lush on the other hand suggests a positive image to the subconscious and healing, rejuvenating energy is directed to the ovaries (or wherever is appropriate to the individual).

Knowledge about the power of the word is supplemented by the awareness that every human being has three basic psychological needs. According to Dr. Cody (2006) those needs are: safety, approval, and control. Depending on our backgrounds, one of these will be prominent. Our psychological need influences the way we speak, the words we choose. When we identify our core need, we can heal it by balancing it at the subconscious level.

In *Revenge of the Wounded Child* (2006) Dr. Cody Horton states that people who continually experience drama in relationships; individuals who simply cannot keep friends for any length of time; or are always trying to find people to identify with, relate to or be accepted by are seeking approval (Horton, 2006). A crisis occurs every time this person's life seems to be going smoothly and puts him at least temporarily at the center of attention—this is also need for approval. A person who is constantly bragging, cheating on a partner, is highly competitive, is always playing *one-upmanship* is seeking approval. According to Dr. Horton (2006) financial instability (I'm not good enough, I don't deserve it) and *why does this always happen to me?* also stem straight from lack of approval. She calls this phenomenon the *Approval Trance*.

With the *Control Trance* we find individuals who always need to be right, who are controlling and manipulative, who are highly critical of others, are outwardly oppositional even if they secretly agree with you, and who monopolize the conversation. They actually feel inferior, vulnerable, and out of control but their behaviors create for them an illusion of safety. Many of these people would like to be a real part of what is going on around them but their lack of confidence makes it difficult for them. Their unresolved woundedness causes them to feel insecure and inadequate; desperately afraid of being perceived as weak these types expend masses of energy trying to protect themselves through their control façade (Horton, 2006).

To feel safe we feel we must have complete, absolute and total knowledge. We watch the news, we scour the internet, we check the *Farmer's Almanac*, and we pursue various modalities. Unfortunately you can find validation for pretty much anything you want if you look long enough and with the internet it is just not that difficult. The problem is that the conflicting information then undermines the safety we seek to acquire and we end up feeling confused and frightened all over again—perhaps more than before. News reports and even some television commercials use the hypnotic trigger of fear to get us to tune in, to listen to what they have to say. We do because we are desperately seeking safety so a vicious cycle results. Dr. Horton (2006) calls this the *Safety Trance*.

We all have safety, control or approval needs; we may even recognize more than one in ourselves. Recognition is key—the way I explain it to clients is that recognizing or acknowledging when you have an issue(s) is like shining a bright flashlight into a dark corner, the shadows disappear and you can see things clearly. If we don't deal with our shadow it will most definitely deal with us. What we won't express, what we refuse, suppress, ignore, deny, or hide will not be denied. The power of the word—the power of the subconscious mind—are yours for the taking, the application, the acceptance, the knowing, the benefit, the healing . . . the unfolding of your fertility journey.

Dr. Brian Weiss states that not one single problem can possibly be solved until awareness of it bubbles up into consciousness (2000). Dr. Weiss says that we are all physicians of the soul and so in our daily dealings and healings we must come from the heart; the true heart, not the head. If at any time we are in doubt, Dr. Weiss recommends that we follow our hearts. This does not mean to deny your own empirical experiences but rather that you are to trust yourself to integrate intuition and experience. Dr. Weiss suggests we would do well to nurture the balance and harmony between the head and the heart. As I have said, Dr. Weiss also states that the more you practice listening to intuition: that calm inner voice or "gut feeling," and the more you trust, the more accurate and clear the voice will become (2000).

The awareness of these psychological needs (be they our own or those of others) and the ability to utilize words effectively enables us to more efficiently navigate the world we live in. Clear understanding of our own process—as well as the processes of others—significantly reduces stress and provides us with great insight, which, in turn, allows us to better express ourselves, and our needs, and to communicate with others.

Chapter 21

HOLDING THE SPACE

"Trees are the earth's endless effort to speak to the listening heaven."

—*Rabindranath Tagore*

What I feel my work really comes down to is holding the space for my clients' healing. My initial session is two hours and a good part of it is listening. I listen to women who have not been heard, perhaps in a long time, perhaps ever. Not only do I listen, but I hear. And I validate what has been done, what is going on with women in these situations. Oftentimes dealing with infertility has put a serious strain on a relationship. Husbands are sometimes overwhelmed by the constant emotional havoc—his wife's grief, her self-hatred or blame, her high anxiety as she tries to micromanage the process and make something happen. He doesn't know what to do or say, and he may well feel helpless. She can have a broad range of emotions and feeling inept and disempowered she may rapidly run the gamut without even realizing it.

A lot of times wives become frustrated with their husbands because women tend to be verbal processors while men are often not. He may feel a subject has been completely covered in a few sentences or in a short talk. She, on the other hand, may think he doesn't care because he doesn't like to go over all the details repeatedly or because he processes more quickly and has come to terms with the situation before she has even grasped it. Seeing me takes the pressure off both husband and wife: I provide the listening and validation she needs and can also be objective in the assessment of what her husband is "really" thinking.

The bottom line is that men and women are different. They have different brains, they process information differently. Most men do not have the emotional wherewithal to withstand the crushing weight of the years of tests, cyclic disappointments, ovulation predictors, timed intercourse, fertility drugs, IUIs, premature talk about donor eggs, negative prognoses, repeated IVFs, genetic concerns, financial upsets, and so much more that is the fertility journey. The worst of it is they really can't deal with the mental, emotional, and even physical pain it is causing their wives.

According to Dr. Judith Herman (1997), author of *Trauma and Recovery,* during the late nineteenth century the disorder known as hysteria became a prime focus of serious medical inquiry. Because the term *hysteria* was so commonly understood at that time, no one had actually taken the time to systematically define it. Basically, as one historian put it, "for twenty-five centuries, hysteria had been considered a strange disease with incoherent and incomprehensible symptoms. Most physicians believed it to be a disease proper to women and originating in the uterus" (p. 10). Incidentally, the word hysteria comes from the Greek word for uterus. Another historian explained that hysteria was "a dramatic medical metaphor for everything that men found mysterious or unmanageable in the opposite sex" (p. 10).

Hypnosis was one of the most effective tools applied to hysteria in the early days. Unfortunately, the issue and the methods to treat it were not well understood and eventually many efforts to work with hysteria were abandoned. Another reason is because the men who were conducting the research couldn't fathom the sheer amount of abuse women had endured in those days and chose to deny the truth. I could go deep into discussion about this topic—women having endured real trauma were often dismissed or discounted; their anguish trivialized and untreated as they were labeled hysteric. However, I included the paragraph because—especially in the fertility industry—we still see the discounting and denying of women's feelings and needs. What women dealt with hundreds of years ago still occurs. Thankfully, we know it and we know how to take care of it.

Many of my clients have no one to talk to. They recognize that it is stressing their husbands but they have no one else. They may have friends or parents or sisters but these people may not understand or sympathize and may do more harm than good with their insensitive comments. Support groups are not particularly conducive to the infertility topic because as people in the support group become pregnant they leave the group. Those who are among the last feel abandoned, feel "less than" the others, feel they are being punished; those who do conceive early on may experience a form of survivors' guilt. Once women become pregnant they typically have little or no desire to stay around people still dealing with infertility. Clients still waiting to become pregnant don't tend to see the other pregnancies as inspiring.

Online groups concern me and I said so in *It's Conceivable!* I get lots of referrals from online groups and blogs and I am eternally grateful, however because the subconscious mind responds powerfully to emotion and does not recognize the difference between "reality" and "imagination" it is unable to distinguish someone else's experience from your own. For example, if you are in an online group with twelve women waiting to do IVF and four out of the first six fail before you have had your turn you have now gone through a mental rehearsal of four failed IVFs and two successful ones. As negative emotions are stronger than positive ones the failed IVFs will effectively blot out the successes in your mind. The subconscious is goal-achieving; it easily follows directions like one would follow a blueprint. Because the subconscious is non-logical, and non-thinking, it does not question the idea that the failed IVFs were not physically yours. You go for your

IVF with the worst case scenario in the forefront of your subconscious mind.

As virtually all of my clients are Type-A personalities or have perfectionist tendencies and such, I have no doubt you will understand this analogy. If you've ever had to give a talk, teach a class, do some kind of high pressure business presentation, have your skills somehow evaluated, you know that one negative evaluation can easily knock out 100 positives. You are probably nodding your head right now—that's what my clients do when I bring up this point. You may know that someone has it out for you, and you may know that the people in charge realize that and have even told you not to worry. You have 99 top score evaluations and you brood over the one negative one for days or even longer.

This is an easy and even familiar issue that we can relate to. This illuminates clearly for us just how powerful a negative suggestion—even if it's relatively minor—can be compared to a positive (or 99 positives even if they are absolutely glowing). If we can be hit that hard over something that we logically know has nothing to do with us (if there are 99 positives and 1 negative, it's *that* person, not you!), what impact does negative versus positive IVF results have?

This is what we call an imprint on the subconscious mind. Whether you have had multiple negative IVFs, miscarriages, etc. or whether you have been emotionally invested in someone else's experience doesn't matter. Subconscious imprints must be removed—they are one of the top causes of unexplained infertility I have found in my practice. This is why I have chosen to utilize the power of hypnosis in my profession. People don't always understand what hypnosis really is which is why I wrote *It's Conceivable!*

In a nutshell, guided imagery, creative visualization, and guided meditation are pieces of hypnosis. They are effective for certain issues, but these techniques do not address hypnosis/relaxation depth levels; the needs of various people's personalities to have certain kinds of induction methods; how to purge the subconscious mind of negative thoughts, beliefs, and perceptions; how to heal the psyche; how to positively impact the central nervous system; how to utilize the power of the autonomic nervous system; or how to do hypnotic regression, gestalt or inner world rebuilding.

Hypnosis is more powerful than the various pieces I mentioned above; those techniques are helpful and healing but I prefer having them *and* more. The big guns if you will. The best definition of hypnosis I have ever found is: the bypass of the critical faculty (also called factor) of the mind. Everything I do is designed to achieve this first and foremost. Without the bypass we have nothing.

The critical faculty can be bypassed by hypnotic induction, startle/fear, relaxation, or boredom. Therapeutic hypnotic induction is what occurs in my office and on the personal recordings I make for my distance clients. Hypnotherapists can induce hypnosis with a startle technique (that is usually reserved for stage hypnotism), and that is exactly the technique used by doctors, medical professionals or others (often inadvertently) who deliver bad news (you have less than 1% chance of pregnancy even with IVF) that shocks you; and while you are in this vulnerable (emotion = language of the subconscious mind) state they deliver a direct suggestion (you need to do donor egg and immediately, you have no time to spare!).

It is the bypass of the critical faculty—and only the bypass of the critical faculty—that allows negative suggestions and imprints to be removed via the appropriate hypnotic technique. I determine the right technique by evaluating my client and her situation. I start with a foundation and I build on it. To set the stage I tell my clients a story of an overflowing teacup that comes from a Zen proverb: a philosopher visits a Zen Master for tea. The Master pours the tea until it overflows the cup, and just keeps pouring.

The philosopher finally yells for the Master to stop pouring because the tea is overflowing, spilling everywhere, and there is no room for anymore. The Zen Master responds that this is exactly so, that when we are filled with our own fears, opinions, blocks, and so forth we are unable to receive, we are unable to learn, we are unable to take in the new. This is a powerful maxim that inevitably causes a metaphorical light bulb to spark. Describing this scenario I am able to clearly express how the time my client spends talking with me serves to empty her cup and provide space to do the necessary work. In other words, we have room to pour.

I consider myself to be an enlightened witness; this is a term I first encountered in the works of trauma psychologist Alice Miller. An enlightened witness, by my interpretation of the expression, basically validates (without judgment) the pain and trauma another human being has experienced and helps them to transcend it so they can heal in all areas of their lives. The support of a true enlightened witness is essential to success; acknowledgement, acceptance, and validation of the grave impact of infertility upon human lives are crucial.

I have, as I mentioned in Chapter 14, likened the infertility diagnosis to that of catastrophic illness—with the exception that it gets none of the social support or recognition made available to sufferers of cancer, etc. I believe this is an important comparison to make, as the dismissal of an individual's crisis only serves to exacerbate it. Healing begins in recognition—you cannot proceed without it. I believe this is the reason the so-called infertility epidemic has progressed to its present level; its emotional effects are so often discounted. My own individual cognizance—concrete experience combined with empathy, energy, and intuition—enables me to effectively utilize hypnotherapeutic fertility applications, and helped form the foundation of the *Spirit Baby Whisperer* work I do today.

The initial session, during which as I mentioned I spend a good deal of time listening to what my client has to share with me, is also my intake and provides me with much of what I need to know to set up a treatment plan of sorts. I take thorough notes during client sessions: usually four to six pages on intake. This is because your words are crucial to your success. I use what is virtually a formula that—at its most simplified—is: your words plus my technique equals your success. I know how to impact your subconscious mind most effectively because of the role you play. We are a team, we work together.

Having worked with fertility clients predominantly now for a dozen years, I have come to find that twelve sessions seems to be the "lucky" number. I have had clients conceive after only one session but I've also worked with clients for twenty or thirty before they conceive. These are the extreme ends of the spectrum—on a bell curve they are the outer ends. I've come to suggest twelve sessions so that I have enough time to do the necessary work; it's not fair to the process if someone comes in only once, doesn't conceive, and blames the hypnosis. Though I have psychic input, I am not simply reading my clients, I am not just telling you whether you will or will not have a baby. I am working with you to bring your baby into this world in just the right time and in just the right way and I need the time to do it.

I started out recommending four to six sessions and saying that it might take more or less. This is what you will find in *It's Conceivable!* My clients are committed to bringing their babies into the world and they realize there is a lot of baggage or trauma or stress to be dealt with. I have not even had to become selective as to whom I accept into my practice as the Universe seems to have done that for me: the clients who come to me are there for a reason.

The purpose of the work I do is to help you to get your life back first and foremost. The baby is actually the icing on the cake. In order to get pregnant there is a balance that must be attained: that is the balance of intention and surrender. Let go and let God. You cannot left brain a baby but you can't simply dream one up either. You must put the intention out there, you must wish, but beyond that you must ask. Put it out to the Universe, pray to God/dess. Then you figure out what you can do such as doing your hypnosis, meditating, taking supplements, going to doctor appointments, etc. You do what you can do and you surrender the rest. This balance must be achieved for pregnancy to occur. I can actually see/sense this when it occurs in people; there is an energy shift that is quite perceptible.

There are three keys to conception and they contain all of the steps I have been speaking of. They are simple, yet powerful, and following them will enable you to get your life back; to achieve balance of mind, body, and spirit; to achieve balance of intention and surrender; and to create the correct energy vibration that aligns you with your spirit baby and basically serves as an attractor beam. I was given these keys nearly twenty years ago as I prepared to bring my second son into the world.

The first key is to meditate. To go into the silence where you are closer to God, to Goddess, to Source, to Spirit, to Creator . . . Hypnosis is the easiest way to do this, particularly for those who have trouble quieting their minds. Hypnosis has a rapid effect on the mind and impacts the mind/body/spirit as meditation does, as is it complementary to various meditation techniques. For our intents and purposes here hypnosis and meditation are interchangeable for daily practice.

The second key is to listen. Meditation helps to develop the intuition, and through the hypnotic process we are reconnecting you to innate abilities such as intuition, natural conception, rejuvenation and regeneration. Once you are spending regular time in the field of intention (as Deepak Chopra calls it), in silence, with God, in Source, with the Creator . . . you will be receiving pertinent information to the conception of your baby. Now, you must listen. You know what you need to do or not do; it is vital that you listen. And continue to meditate. It is often said that prayer is when you talk to God; meditation is when God talks to you. Listen.

The third key is to trust. Have you ever received intuitive guidance and not listened? And then wished you had have listened? Or you listened but refused to trust, to believe that what you were getting was right. I often tell my clients that if their husbands are looking particularly attractive to them or they smell really good all of a sudden then to have sex by all means. Even if it isn't the right time of the month, even if they are getting ready to meet with a reproductive specialist, and even if it doesn't seem logical. Once you have been having hypnotherapy, practicing hypnosis/meditation every day, and begun listening to your intuition, you will receive conception information and you must trust it!

I received these three keys from my guide and I used them to bring my baby son into the world. I took a meditation/hypnosis class and practiced the guided journeys every day. The instructor of the classes had us do exercises to connect with our inner guides. We accomplished this through hypnosis and automatic writing. Automatic writing is a popular and effective uncovering technique that can be used to find lost items; remember things you've long forgotten; to release subconscious blocks; and to communicate with guides, angels, as well as your own subconscious mind.

Many of the other students' guides were much chattier than mine. Mine started out by giving me a one word message: meditate. Over and over my guide would direct my hand to write the word: meditate. So I meditated. I enjoyed it and it was part of the class anyway. After a few weeks my guide finally gave me a new word: listen. I found this more confusing than the word meditate, but I continued with my meditation and simply paid attention to what was happening around me, to what people said, to what I read, and so forth. My intuition became stronger, and I felt more in tune with the Universe in general. I received the third word, trust, sometime before I conceived my baby. I trusted, and I conceived. I just knew one day that it was the right day; I knew I had conceived, I knew my baby was coming. I meditated, I listened, I trusted.

Chapter 22

MY BABY IS COMING SOON

"If you do not hope, you will not find what is beyond your hopes."

—*St. Clement of Alexandra*

As my spirit baby contacts become more frequent and of greater strength, I continue to note my observations so that I can more effectively understand them. While I am talking to their moms, the spirit babies tend to sit to their mothers' right. That seems to indicate the baby is coming very soon. Other babies are often flying around above their mothers' heads. To me, that means they are coming, but work needs to be done with Mom first. Often while I am hypnotizing my clients their babies will hover over their mothers' bellies or around her face. I can tell if I say something they really like because they expand and glow more brightly. That is the best possible confirmation I could ever hope to get as far as being on track.

I don't always see the babies, I also sense them. This tends to happen a lot with my phone and Skype clients, though sometimes I see them either around the computer screen, or right in my house. I do most of my Skype/phone clients in my home office because it can get kind of hectic at the office, and then there are phone and internet complications more frequently there because there are just more people using them.

People ask what happens if I don't see a baby. I don't make any decision based on that because spirit babies are not static and they are free little souls who can fly happily around as they wish. Usually they will make an appearance if I ask them to though not always when and where I might expect. Also, I may get a knowing that the spirit baby is present—this tends to be the way I receive the baby's (intended) gender.

Occasionally there is a client who decides she doesn't want to get pregnant or have a family. I have not seen this occur very often, maybe three or four times in twelve years. They are happy when they finally admit to themselves what they truly want. This is not a bad thing; some people don't want to experience the role of mother in this lifetime. I always say that the baby is the icing on the cake—the main point of HF is to get your life back. Once you have your life back, once you have that overall balance intact, then you can do what's right for you.

Sometimes women are frightened to read the words of the above paragraph. Those words are not for you. It's frightening, I know, to embark on this journey, particularly with what you've already been through. That is why the work is important, so that such words don't strike fear into your heart. I address the question because some people do ask. I will never write you off, I will never make a decision for you or tell you what to do; I will hold the space for you, and support your process. Sometimes decisions have to be made: use medical intervention, stick with natural conception, donor eggs, donor embryos, adoption . . . from a state of balance, from a place of surrender, you'll be quite amazed how calmly you can consider or discuss these possibilities.

As I've said before, I provide support for my clients. I also provide hope. I spoke to a new client just the other day who told me that she'd thought she had lost all hope until she talked to me. Our first conversation served to rejuvenate her, to let her know—as she put it—that someone actually really cares about her. She has two months until her embryo transfer—we are both thrilled that she has time to connect with her baby, and do whatever work her own process deems necessary to ensure the most positive outcome.

I believe it is because spirit babies guide their parents (usually their mothers) to me that I have seen such amazing success. A client of mine sent me a text yesterday to let me know how smoothly her donor egg embryo transfer had gone. I congratulated her and said I'd received input on three other babies in the same day: one to confirm I was right—the baby's a boy, and one to announce she is thirteen weeks pregnant with twins. My client and I jokingly called it "a very baby day."

I am blessed to have a lot of "very baby days" and I feel that each of my clients energetically supports the others. And it is the energy of the work that is so important. Exceptional hypnotic skill is a necessity, but compassion, intelligence, intuition, professionalism, and positive energy are the qualities to look for in a therapist.

Chapter 23

BALANCING SIGNS

*"The best and most beautiful things in the world
cannot be seen nor touched but are felt in the heart."*

—*Helen Keller*

A couple of years ago a woman came in to see me. She said she was planning to undergo IVF and she only had one shot; she and her husband just couldn't afford to do it again if it didn't work the first time. I did my standard intake and gleaned some important personal information from my client (we'll call her Sharon) that I would weave into my work: her personal sessions. One question I always ask clients during their intake is if they are okay with having multiples. If they want twins, for example, I can include that in the process— because I know the intricate workings of the subconscious mind I know just how to work this in. If they don't want multiples I have to address that immediately or the fear will sabotage what might otherwise be success.

Sharon was eager to get started and excited when I told her that I, her doctor, and her acupuncturist if she decided to use one would be her team, and that we would all be doing our best to support her throughout the next several weeks and even beyond. As it turned out, Sharon's answer to my multiple question was yes as long as everyone would be healthy. I was happy to oblige and her first session set the stage for the weekly sessions we would be doing during her IVF journey. She wasn't too far from the transfer when she first came in so we did have quite a bit of work to do in less time than usual. We worked with both of our schedules so that we could fit her in more than once per week when necessary.

Following her transfer, Sharon came in for what I consider the crucial appointment: between-transfer-and-pregnancy test when the stressor hormones are just straining to break loose into your body and wreak havoc on implantation. She also had an appointment scheduled for pregnancy-test-results-day. On that day she excitedly told me the news: it's positive! As so many women do, Sharon decided to keep working with me through at least the first trimester; she was quite happy with the work and felt reassured each time she came for a session.

One day Molly got a distress call from Sharon: her pregnancy symptoms had "all gone away." Molly performed a superhuman trick or two with the schedule so we could get Sharon right in. Sharon told me what was happening and I told her that often women feel like they've lost their symptoms but it doesn't mean they're no longer pregnant. This situation occurs frequently with pregnancy but for women who have been dealing with infertility it can be devastating no matter how many people tell them it can actually be quite common. It was this way for Sharon too.

I "sensed" into the situation and I told her that I could see and feel spirit babies and what I was getting was that she had a choice as to how many she wanted. At that Sharon dried her tears and with a sniffle repeated what she had said earlier: that she wanted more than one if it would be safe for mother and babies. We did a soothing, healing session and I reiterated Sharon's wish to the babies (not that they hadn't heard) and checked in on them. Within a couple of days we had word from the doctor that Sharon was, indeed, still pregnant.

And not long after that Sharon came in for her session with big, big news. Not only was she pregnant with multiples, she was pregnant with triplets! So much for thinking she wasn't pregnant we laughed. Sharon and I and the babies (two boys and a girl) continued to do sessions in the office until she was put on bed rest. We continued working together by phone utilizing the power of hypnosis to help her to keep the babies in as long as possible, and addressing whatever other issues came up.

A client of mine who worked with me about ten years ago and had triplets keeps me updated from time to time. She swears that the hypnosis is what enabled her to continue her pregnancy as long as she did, for her babies to beat the national standards across the board (as she put it) and to have no developmental or learning issues at all. I have no doubt it will be the same for Sharon and her babies. The triplet clients I've had over the years have done very well and occasionally we'll receive an update.

I will mention here that hypnosis is one of the most effective modalities for preventing pre-term birth in any case—multiples or otherwise. Above and beyond fertility, hypnosis can deal with virtually every pregnancy and birth issue you can imagine: placenta previa, breech turn, shortened cervix, morning sickness (Princess Kate used hypnosis for just this reason), anxiety, birthing, cesarean section preparation and recovery, lactation, and more. Just a couple of weeks ago I prevented a c-section and facilitated the natural vaginal birth the woman wanted—she was not my client, I'd never met her, and I did it by phone. I have done these things myself in my office and on the phone, and I have taught more than 600 therapists worldwide how to apply these methods themselves. Always remember that help is available!

Chapter 24

WOMEN'S RHYTHMS IN HARMONY WITH THE
RHYTHMS OF THE UNIVERSE

*"Religion is about creation, and for that reason religion
should be about the earth."*

—Laurie Cabot

I focus a lot on balance of mind, body, and spirit in healing fertility. Somewhat of an offshoot to this aspect is called Sympathetic Magick. (I use the k here to distinguish the magick referred to in women's circles and by Goddess based spirituality from the mainstream magic attributed to magicians.) Women's rhythms in harmony with the rhythms of the Universe: cycles in time with the moon; energy in harmony with the earth resonance frequency; the deep, fertile earth and the rich, nurturing womb.

In this way we tap into ancient fertility rites. Intrinsic, feminine based knowing that spans eons of human existence; that is archetypically recognized by the very cells of our beings; and that drives us into the arms of the Goddess; of Gaia, the Earth Mother, who will share her wisdom with us if only we would ask. How may we ask?

Tying into ancient times, Marion Woodman tells us of the Black Madonna who is recognized by many religions. The thunder, perfect mind, her wisdom—encompassing, unfathomable—is revealed in the ancient text (Woodman, 1985). A woman, says Woodman, once purging has occurred, often dreams of a black goddess who becomes her bridge between spirit and body. One aspect of the Goddess Sophia, the image of the black goddess opens a woman to the mystery of life being enacted right inside her own body.

While Mary, Woodman illustrates, provides a focus for the "steeliest asceticism, she is also the ultimate of fertility symbols" (Woodman, 1985, p. 122). In loving the abandoned child within herself—which we know is essential not only to balance but to overall healing—a woman becomes pregnant with herself. The beautiful Black Madonna is this: nature impregnated by spirit, the acceptance of the human body as the chalice of the spirit (Woodman, 1985). Redemption of matter, intersection of sexuality and spirituality, the Black Madonna is "the loving biological tie to the body, fertility, babies" (Woodman, 1985, p. 122).

Centuries ago peasants would plant their crops and perform abundance rituals to ensure a plentiful harvest. This is Sympathetic Magick. Straddling broomsticks the farm folk would hop or jump into the air as high as possible, intending for the crops to emulate the energetic action. Whether this helped the farmers with their harvest is irrelevant. The ritual helped the peasants to align with the desired results, and rituals such as the one described here are powerful ways to impact the subconscious mind.

The subconscious mind is the bigger part of the mind; it is the part that always wins when the two parts are in conflict. Various schools of psychology divide the mind into other categories however, for our purposes here we need only use the two: subconscious and conscious. The subconscious mind can be likened to the old brain or the lizard brain in that it handles what we don't need to think about: our reactions, our emotions, the intricacies of our internal systems and organs. It beats our hearts, breathes, blinks our eyes, and swallows for us.

It is through impacting the subconscious mind with effective hypnotic technique that adjustments in hormone levels do happen; that follicle stimulation is able to be enhanced; that healthy embryos are secured and, therefore, not pitched out of the uterus; that miscarriages can be avoided; that nausea and vomiting during pregnancy (NVP) can be relieved; that an incompetent cervix can be supported, if not lengthened; that a placenta previa can be shifted; that a breech baby can be turned, and so much more. I have literally spent tens of thousands of hours in clinical practice; I have facilitated these things, and more. I not only know they are possible, I know they happen. And babies come into this world when it seems it is impossible, when it seems all hope is gone, when it seems it was never meant to be.

Some simple but powerful Sympathetic Magick you can do to draw your baby to you is to create a baby altar. That is, a sacred space where you can put something or a few things to remind your subconscious mind that you want to have a baby (this works for adoption too, and IVF, etc.). A tiny pair of booties will work nicely, an egg, a picture of a baby, a rattle or other baby toy, are just a few examples. Some women have a family heirloom such as a fertility egg, a letter between grandparents, the medallion of a saint, a piece of jewelry, a statue of the Divine Mother—anything that has been passed down and around will powerfully impress the subconscious mind.

In speaking with a client in my office one day a few years ago I mentioned the very topic I have just discussed here. About halfway through the conversation a light bulb suddenly went on for her and she shouted, "The fertility letter!" Apparently, my client's great aunt had written a letter to her mother announcing the impending birth of her first child. The mother had kept the letter and it had eventually ended up in the hands of various family members. As one after the other got pregnant, the letter became the family's pregnancy guarantee.

My client realized that her sister had had the letter a couple of years earlier and had conceived her children. She declared that she would send for the letter immediately. Within a few weeks my client was pregnant. We had done about a half dozen sessions by the time the letter arrived, and we continued to work together as she had a lot to work on. She also felt it was best for the baby to continue on through the first trimester of the pregnancy and then on an "as-need" basis after that.

Another example of Sympathetic Magick is the ancient practice of planting during the new moon. The idea here is that the moon is dark and just beginning to grow full. This symbolically implies growth, and with pregnancy there is literally the imagery of the dark and then tiny sliver of the moon waxing fuller and fuller day by day. Just as the uterus grows bigger as it prepares to nurture a baby from conception to birth. The moon affects the tides, and the moon affects us. (Just ask any emergency room personnel, police officers, psychiatric hospital staff, or obstetrics doctors and nurses who are overwhelmed every time there is a full moon.)

Green is the symbolic color of fertility, and burning a green candle (having it on your altar is a thought) energetically impacts the Universe and your body/mind/spirit with the desire to create, attract, manifest your baby. Burning the candle in accordance with the new to full moon cycle enhances the power of the ritual, as does burning the green candle on one of the three fertility power days: February 2nd (the Goddess fertility day, Imbolc), March 21st-*ish*, the Spring Equinox (the Goddess fertility day, Ostara *aka Easter*), and May 1st (the Goddess fertility day, Beltane). Spring is traditionally the time for fertility, and if any of the above dates coincide with your personal fertility journey it is easy enough to take advantage of them.

For those of you whose fertility journey does not happen to be occurring in the spring, there are other power days as well that span the rest of the calendar year: June 21st which is summer solstice, August 1st (called Lammas), September 21st which is the autumn equinox, October 31st/November 1st (called Samhain and considered the beginning/end of a year's cycle), and December 21st which is the winter solstice. You can still use the green candle or you may choose to use orange. Orange is an attractor color and also coincides with the second chakra, the energy center that governs the reproductive organs and the energy of creativity.

I, myself, was conceived around Spring Equinox; I was born shortly after Winter Solstice. I have always been in alignment with these energies and I believe that I was conceived and born at these times so that I could have the firsthand energetic experience and thus be able to easily pass it along when needed. Perhaps this experience was for me an encoded key designed to activate the appropriate spiritual knowledge—the *Spirit Baby Whisperer* knowledge—when the time was right, the energies aligned.

Lynsi Eastburn

"The image of the Goddess inspires women to see ourselves as divine,
our bodies as sacred,
the changing phases of our lives as holy, our aggression as healthy,
our anger as purifying,
and our power to nurture and create—
but also to limit and destroy when necessary—
as the very force that sustains life.
Through the Goddess, we can discover our strength,
enlighten our minds, own our bodies, and celebrate our emotions.
We can move beyond narrow, constricting roles and become whole."

—*Starhawk*
The Spiral Dance
Chop Wood Carry Water (1984)

Chapter 25

NOAH

"Great men are they who see that spiritual is stronger than any material force—that thoughts rule the world."

—*Ralph Waldo Emerson*

A few months ago I had phone sessions lined up all day and then was scheduled to go over to my office to meet with two more clients. Early in the day I was doing some type of mindless task, straightening up the house or perhaps washing dishes, when I heard the name Noah very clearly in my head. Noah? I don't know anyone named Noah, I thought, as I went about my business. I heard the name again, very clearly, but inside my head. Noah? I don't know any Noah's I mused as I made a mental run through of any of my clients who had any kids (occasionally my clients do have kids as we are working with secondary infertility). Still no Noahs. Well, I figured, maybe it's one of the new babies.

As I spoke to my clients I mentioned the name, Noah, to see if it held any meaning to them. Absolutely nothing—just didn't resonate with anybody. I just let it go; I assumed I'd find out what it was about when I was supposed to. The next day I, again, had several phone clients scheduled. One was with a client who was 38 weeks pregnant and having contractions. We hadn't been sure she'd even be able to keep the appointment but as it turned out she could. Not long after the call began my client mentioned that she needed to pick a name for her baby. Instantly, I heard a jangling in my head of Noah! Noah! Noah! Noah! Noah! I pushed it aside figuring that nobody was interested yesterday and I don't want this woman to feel like I'm trying to influence her choice.

My client said she was going to list some names to discuss with her husband that evening and, again, I heard the insistent Noah! Noah! Noah! Noah! Noah! Noah! Noah! I also heard a voice tell me to tell her, and that Noah is connected to her husband. I sighed and told my client, "I'm just going to toss this out there, I have no attachment to it: Noah." She laughed and said that was the name her husband wanted to name the baby and they had just talked to someone about that name. I told her about the Noah yammering in my head and we joked that this baby (a boy) seemed to really want that name. We left it at that and I stopped hearing the distracting shrieks of Noah! in my head. About two weeks later my office received an e-mail asking my assistants to, "Please tell Lynsi that Noah was born (date/time/particulars) . . . she'll understand the message."

I am able to see spirit babies and I am able to hear them. I am also able to feel their presence, and just cognitively know they are there. Different experiences at different times. I usually don't need to hear anybody as clearly as Noah; the hypnosis work we do together helps you to better hear/see/sense/know your baby. Noah's mother is a very busy physician and had also experienced some serious trauma. In this case it was easier for the baby to communicate through me and through his father. Note here that he *did* get his message across.

Chapter 26

DAMAGE CONTROL

"No one can make you feel inferior without your consent."

—*Eleanor Roosevelt*

I often talk about damage control and I have recently decided to focus my entire talk on that aspect of HypnoFertility® at an event for hypnotherapists to whom I've been invited to speak in Las Vegas. I've done a lot of what I call damage control over the years, much of it in cleaning up after uninformed hypnotherapists. This may sound a bit harsh but there are many people practicing hypnobirthing or other such techniques that have not taken hypnotherapy training and are relying on a syllabus and/or written scripts to work with clients. I end up with their traumatized clients in my office (or on the phone) and I have to undo what has so carelessly been done.

This happens with other professionals as well, and with the general public. It bothers me most, though, when it's someone who should know better: hypnotic languaging, waking hypnosis, painted words, and impact on the subconscious mind, etc. The average person wouldn't be expected to know all that, but a hypnotist of even the lowest caliber should. On the bright side, I can release trauma caused by insensitive and even cruel remarks that breeze by the critical faculty and cause the formation of subconscious blocks. What has been done can be undone by a properly trained therapist.

Years ago, I had a client come into town to see me and to visit one of the Denver-area reproductive clinics. She had been traveling back and forth, and had elected to come to the Denver clinic originally because she wanted to work with me and we were both located in the same area. I worked with her in office and by phone. One weekend she came into town and had booked a session with me. At my office she asked me if I could recommend an acupuncturist. I said I would call to get a referral near where she was staying but as it turned out, by the time I had the number for her she had already found someone to try. A couple of days later my client, an MD with a highly regarded specialty, came in and told me about the horror she had experienced with this acupuncturist.

First of all, the woman got my client on the table and then, while my client was lying there with needles protruding from every which way, proceeded to ask my client if she wasn't scared to do IVF? The acupuncturist had, she told my client, done it once herself, and it was "such a horror" that she decided not to do it ever again. She decided to remain childless. My client told me she had begun the cancel, cancel technique the minute the negativity began spewing from the so-called healer, and that she had used it well over a hundred times in this acupuncturist's office. She was very grateful to have had the technique so she could do some damage control herself, preventing the insensitive, unprofessional, and inappropriate (if not unethical) words of the acupuncturist from seeping into her soul. That day we had to focus the session on clearing that horrendous episode.

A contact that I work with at one of the reproductive clinics told me some time ago that they were going to have to remove one of their acupuncturists from their referral list. The woman had been a nurse prior to becoming an acupuncturist (this is actually quite common) and had begun to let her Western medicine ideas intrude upon patient sessions. An acupuncturist is there to be an acupuncturist, and he/she should not be giving you Western medicine advice: that's for your reproductive endocrinologist to do. No acupuncturist should be telling you your eggs are no good, or that the doctor shouldn't be allowing you to do IVF. That is the doctor's decision—the doctor's and yours (and your partner). If you don't trust your doctor, then by all means get another one, but don't pay a specialist all that money to listen to someone who has no business giving you Western medical advice.

I have had some clients encounter inconsiderate medical personnel including nurses and doctors, and also embryologists. Recently, a client was on the table awaiting her embryo transfer: she had one frozen, four cell embryo but she was in good spirits. Until the embryologist walked in, looked at the embryo, and said, "I'm sorry." If the clinic has elected to do the procedure then this type of input is totally unnecessary and unhelpful.

One nurse looked at another of my client's embryos and told my client she couldn't understand why the doctor was even bothering. Well, the doctor *is* bothering so why would you say anything to the contrary? That is down and out ego and it has no place in this process. There is a saying: *if you have nothing good to say, don't say anything at all.* Truer words were never spoken; however, since very few people seem to adhere to that adage, I have my hands full with damage control.

Simply entering a fertility clinic can subject you to potential emotional damage. One clinic has a reputation for practically insisting that their patients do donor eggs. The issue isn't the donor eggs, it's that these people are usually not ready to jump that far ahead and have had no time to process such an unexpected direction. Many times women go into a fertility clinic with the hopes of having some tests run and getting the go-ahead to start trying to conceive naturally. Barring that, there are other options such as Clomid and/or IUIs, and even IVF to be considered before donor eggs. Donor eggs are also, for many women/couples, on par with adoption or choosing to remain childless so it is no wonder women who receive a premature donor egg prognosis feel so shattered. This type of thing happens far too frequently; finding out we can release it brings great relief to such recipients.

We have all heard of the placebo effect; we've heard stories about sugar pills, surgery performed on the wrong knee healing the injured one, drug studies where one group gets a placebo pill rather than the actual drug and does just as well. We can leverage the placebo effect with hypnosis depending on the situation. The nocebo effect (a negative placebo effect, a self-fulfilling prophecy) can be as powerful as the placebo effect, if not more. I tend to lean toward the *more* side as I'm aware just how much harder something negative impacts us than something positive.

Dr. Bruce Lipton validates exactly what I have seen and repeatedly stated for years in my own practice: that both the words and demeanor of a physician can easily convey hope-deflating, frightening, distressing messages that inadvertently convey to you the belief that you are powerless (Lipton, 2005). Dr. Deepak Chopra, Dr. Bernie Siegel, and other medical doctors who regularly integrate mind/body medicine often mention various case studies that identify the phenomenon of patients dying from cancer or other issues they didn't have. This shows us just how strong the power of suggestion can be.

I received a distress call from a woman in Scotland who had been to see one of my own graduate students. She was about to undergo an IVF frozen transfer with two embryos. Not long before the scheduled transfer, the hypnotherapist told the client that she should really just get used to the idea that she wasn't going to have any more children. The woman, who had read *It's Conceivable!,* told the hypnotherapist flat out: Lynsi wouldn't say that! She walked out of the office and telephoned America.

My assistant scrambled to move my appointments around so I could schedule a Skype session with the woman from Scotland. Not easy to do on limited time and with a seven hour time difference! We managed it, however, and I was able to work with the lady to undo what someone who had even taken my training had done. (I can't control those I train, they take their hypnotherapy training elsewhere most times and I can only give them a protocol and teach them to follow it. I can't ensure they will honor it, and I can't control for ego.)

In yet another example, I recently spoke with a client who conceived her baby a year or so ago—the little sweetie slipped right in while Mom was on an IVF waiting list. Feeling the presence of another baby, and wanting another child, my client decided to have a couple more sessions with me. Between our Skype meetings, my client went to a "well-respected" psychic soul reader in her area. The woman told my client that she had karma for multiple pregnancies and that there was a male spirit that didn't come through (due to miscarriage) who was interfering with her energy now. The reader said that sometimes such spirits would think of this type of thing as punishment for her or for himself, and could then come through handicapped.

She told my client that such spirits punish the mothers by being handicapped or out of alignment. The soul reader then gave her a meditation to do to clear the interference. A couple of months later my client went back for a follow-up session. The woman told her that she was now fine, and that her creative talent is to have babies. However, the woman advised my client that, "I wouldn't take a chance on getting pregnant again if I were you." She proceeded to tell my client that if she conceives under stress the baby will be handicapped, and that she could have stopped after four pregnancies since, in this woman's view of things, this baby is a choice rather than karmic. Above and beyond all of that confusion, the reader then told my client that if she does IVF she will have twins.

That reading was a chaotic disaster. The back and forth of it is ludicrous—the woman was constantly contradicting herself. My client was seriously distressed—though "emotionally trashed" might actually be a more accurate word choice—because this soul reader apparently has a good reputation; fortunately she knew enough about this type of thing to immediately get in touch with me. I told my client that the woman had been unable to accurately read her (my client is an energy worker and spiritual healer) so this soul reader had allowed ego and personal opinion to color the reading. Even on Skype I could see the damage in my client's aura, and her energy was down significantly. I reinforced what she and I both know about spirit babies, and I proceeded with the necessary clearing and repair post haste.

Virtually every client I have ever met has been traumatized in some similar way to the above examples. The harmful effects of negative suggestions that can damage one's health are the nocebo effect. This is one of the most insidious problems I find myself working with in the fertility world. Simply navigating our own world leaves us open to such experiences; they are more frequent the more we deal with traditional Western medicine, and certainly the more we deal with *in*fertility. Knowing how all of this impacts your subconscious mind arms you with emotional, spiritual, and physical protection. Knowledge is power—this is true. And now you have it.

The issues here are also what we refer to as waking hypnosis. With waking hypnosis the critical faculty is bypassed without formal hypnotic induction. If you consider that emotion is the language of the subconscious mind you can see how effective a statement given to someone in an emotional or vulnerable state can be—this is evidenced in the above examples of the unethical acupuncturist, the soul reader, etc. Ads and commercials are also examples of waking hypnosis— think jingles, for example. Waking hypnosis is a fascinating phenomenon and often used by people who will swear they don't even know what it is, let alone use it. The cancel technique is the best counter for waking suggestion—if a doctor, nurse, embryologist, librarian—whoever—gives you information that is out of harmony with what is essential to your success: CANCEL, CANCEL!

Trust

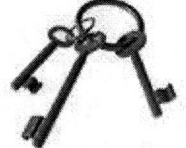

Chapter 27

A KID LIKE THAT

"Our deepest wishes are whispers of our authentic selves. We must learn to respect them. We must learn to listen."

—Sarah Ban Breathnach

My son, Dylan, will tell you he is the first HypnoFertility® baby, and he is right. However, there is another one that occurred not long after Dylan's little baby body had begun growing in my womb. I was born in Toronto, Canada and lived there for the first twenty years of my life. I then bought a house in Kitchener, a city I really enjoyed. My children's dad was in sales/service and back in the early nineties the NAFTA agreement went through and Canada's economy absolutely tanked. You pretty much had to know someone to get a job in a fast food place, and three of the main factories pulled out of Kitchener leaving thousands unemployed in what is basically a blue collar town. Fortunately we were offered a transfer to the United States; with such a bleak outlook we felt we could hardly turn it down. In November 1993 we relocated to Duluth, GA.

Georgia was definite culture shock for me. Trying to get my bearings I found a meditation class to join and it was here that I met my friend, Julie. In getting to know each other we asked the usual questions: are you married, do you have any kids, what do you do . . .? I had a four-year-old son at the time and was not yet pregnant with my youngest. Julie mentioned that she had infertility—nine years of unprotected intercourse—but that they hadn't pursued it too far because she didn't really want kids anyway. I simply said, "Oh." I didn't think much about it, that was her choice and she didn't seem unhappy about it. Julie was 38-years-old at the time.

A couple of months or so later, I met up with Julie and I brought my son, Kelly, with me. Kelly was (and still is) a charmer. Everyone loves him. He's very intelligent; he was such a cute little kid: he was friendly, he could immediately put you at ease, athletic . . . people would stop me at the airport or the mall to tell me he looked like Macaulay Culkin but "cuter" (he was also younger) and an airplane pilot once took his authentic wings off and gave them to Kelly on the spot because he was downright flabbergasted that Kelly knew and could name all the planes in the sky. Julie just loved him.

After we'd gotten together a couple of times Julie made an offhand remark to the effect of: "Well, I would have a kid if it could be like Kelly!" I jokingly responded with, "Oh, you can, you just need to know the formula!" Julie looked at me somewhat in shock (this is a bypass of the critical faculty—waking hypnosis) and I said, "Just read Stephen King books every night before bed and you'll have a baby like him." I was not formally trained in hypnosis at that time and didn't realize how powerful that little exchange had been.

A month or so later, Julie wasn't feeling very well. I could hear the words in my head: she's pregnant! And I knew it was true. After listening to her symptoms and her reiterating several times that she'd never felt like this I said, "Julie, you're pregnant." Of course, the response was, "no I'm not, I can't get pregnant." We ended the conversation with me telling her to get to a doctor. She did; I was right. Julie was just stunned and it took her quite a while to adjust to the news. Since I was already pregnant by then, it was nice we could be pregnant together.

Julie's baby was a little girl born six months after my baby son. Joey, as they called her, was so much like Kelly they could have been related. She was cute and smart, calm and easygoing, she was basically made-to-order. That's actually an important statement. As I was describing Kelly I couldn't help but think how much it sounded like I was bragging. But I wasn't—I was just telling you what he's like. That's what I wanted and that's what I "put out for" prior to conceiving him. My youngest son is very similar—they're not identical but they share so many of the same qualities.

Julie wasn't really infertile; she told me that she didn't want "some little brat" that's running all over the place, screaming in the grocery store, etc. That fear was powerful enough for her subconscious mind to prevent her from becoming pregnant. I, inadvertently, told her subconscious mind that other types of children are possible, and she accepted the suggestion both consciously and subconsciously. This happens a lot. Women have sisters, cousins, friends—even parents—who don't discipline or can't handle their children and they make a decision not to have kids because they don't want those problems. It's not an accurate decision, but the subconscious mind is not logical.

Chapter 28

THE DOORS

"Prayer is not asking. It is a longing of the soul. It is daily admission of one's weakness. It is better in prayer to have a heart without words than words without a heart."

—*Mahatma Gandhi*

Much of the information I have put into HF I came upon intuitively. I have been trained in energy work: Reiki, therapeutic touch, crystal healings. I also have degrees and/or certifications in psychology, gestalt therapy, counseling, hypnotism, meditation, yoga and many others. I have always been a reader (I have an English degree as well) and besides formal education have acquired a great deal of knowledge through self-education. I follow the basic methods I describe to you here to navigate my own life. I meditate, do self-hypnosis, and practice yoga virtually every day. In turn, I listen to my intuition. What to do, where to go, what is my gut telling me? And, probably most important of all, I trust the information.

This is how I became the *Spirit Baby Whisperer*. This is how I found myself working virtually exclusively with fertility clients, developing a method that is now my signature style, teaching therapists, and educating the public on a grand scale as an author. I was guided to do it all; no one set the course for me, I blazed the trail. But not alone, I followed Divine guidance that I could hear because meditative conditioning enabled me to match the frequency, and that I could download because of trust.

I trust the creative process, I trust the Universe. And they get top priority over anything any human being—with his/her eye on nothing but the money—could ever propose. I do my best to surround myself with such people as I know the energies feed each other and in so doing maintain a continuous cleansing and balancing. It creates a positive feedback loop, in essence.

I was guided a few weeks ago to rent a little cabin in the mountains with my husband so that we could both work uninterrupted on our current books. We did it, and we both could tell immediately that we'd made a good choice in doing so. Not only do we have the time and quiet space to write; but also access to nature where we can cleanse our energies; clear our heads; and just absorb the life affirming energies of the trees; wander upon the Earth Mother at leisure; and soak up the ions from the crisp, clear mountain lake.

I was guided to get this book out—and fast. Though I did plan to start working on it, I hadn't been in a hurry. Now, however, it is November 10, 2012 and I have a release date and first book signing scheduled in February 2013. I don't question, I trust; I know it will come to be. When you follow your path, when you listen, things come together beautifully. Prior to being urged to complete this book, I was guided to read/reread three books of spiritual text: *The Baghavad Gita*, *The Upanishads*, and *The Dhammapada*. During meditation I received the name *Tom* across the screen of my mind and the understanding that I was to contact him about meditation. Tom, it turns out, holds a weekly meditation group in a wonderful space at his home. The energy is fantastic; the room is accentuated with some beautiful paintings including one that features Krishna. I personally love the purple wall-to-wall carpet chosen expressly for its divine connection (purple is the color of the crown chakra).

Serendipitously, a yogi from India was leading the first gathering my husband and I attended. He showed me a meditation to work with and I began to practice it immediately. This ties together because Krishna is the God featured in the *Bhagavad Gita* and I had just finished rereading it. *The Gita* tells us that there are doors in the body from which the soul can enter and exit. While working with a client in my office I was shown a vision of just how to do this with a spirit baby; I have incorporated this into my work with remarkable results. Had I not paid attention to my spiritual guidance I would have missed out on learning a revolutionary method for connecting mothers with spirit babies.

Chapter 29

DIVINE MOTHER

"There are many paths to enlightenment.
Be sure to take the one with a heart."

— *Lao Tzu*

Throughout this writing I have tried to express God in
various terms. I know that individual religions tend to have
their absolutes in this regard, but I don't—and I can't if I'm
going to be supportive to all my clients. If a client has a strong
traditional Catholic faith, for example, I ask her how we can
incorporate that into the HF process. Most people who come
to see me, frankly, are not of the single-minded or judgmental
type that people typically think of when thinking of religion. I
am open to spirituality, and to religion, non-judgmentally.

I meditate in many places both at home and at my
office. I have a tiny little space that is basically behind a chair in
my living room that I have taken to lately. I have a few plants
there and a window, and it is just peaceful. Bit by bit I have
accumulated sacred artifacts: first a Buddha with a candle; then
a statue of Ganesha; a picture of Krishna; a beautiful, pale blue
Angelite crystal sphere (represents the angels) that was given to
me by a student; a Divine Mother statue; a tiny Quan Yin, a
Mother Mary candle; etc. I also display a few spiritual books

here as well. It is not necessary to have any of these things in your meditation space, I just happen to enjoy them.

I incorporate the divinity of all traditions as it so decides to reveal itself to me. Seated in my tiny oasis one day in September I was shown a powerful image from the Great Mother. As it happened, I was sitting with my new copy of Clarissa Pinkola Estes' book *Untie the Strong Woman: Blessed Mother's Immaculate Love,* my Mary candle (that happens to be adorned with a picture matching the cover photo of the book), a statue of Quan Yin (known for her fertility properties), and, seated peacefully in the earth at the base of my indoor tree, the Divine Mother. I was thinking how this would be a great time to do a sacred feminine meditation—to just reach for the Goddess and open to her wisdom in the now.

As I sank gently into the joy of my seated meditation, I simply opened myself to the Divine Mother, became receptive to the ancient knowledge she would share with me, the blessings of her love. A phenomenon known as time distortion occurs during deep hypnosis or meditation; it was no different for me at this time. Because the conscious mind is linear, and because the ego likes to measure its accomplishments, we use time during waking, daily life to keep track of various things: appointment times, dates, days of the week, people's ages, etc. In the subconscious mind time (if it exists at all) is more fluid and free. It can speed up or slow down or very pleasantly drift. The past and the future do not exist in the subconscious; everything is happening in the present. Therefore, during deep hypnosis/meditation, the perceived past, present and future blend together into one time, this time, this very moment, now . . . expressed naturally and without question. The subconscious mind simply is *(being)*. The conscious mind tries to distinguish *(doing)*.

Linear time dissolved and I found myself gently bathed in a soothing rose-pink light; the love of the Goddess, the sacred feminine. As though I'd been transported to another dimension—which, perhaps, I had—I suddenly became aware of what can only be described as luscious colors swirling around me, merging with the pink light, twirling, melting, churning in emphasis; patterns, colors rarely glimpsed from the world of solid. In awe, as I can never help but being in this level, I simply let go into receptivity, as had been my intent from the start. My chakras blossomed, aligned fully with Source energy, and from this state of introspective bliss I watched the Divine Mother's message to me unfold.

She appeared, robes of heaven flowing easily around her earthy feminine form; compassionate, wise and strong; designed and patterned; surrounded by dozens of magnificent angels upon the indigo back drop of the stars. It was fascinating to see and incredible to experience; the angels and the Divine Mother weaving blankets of celestial light with a triple knot pattern—a Celtic emblem of the trinity, the triple Goddess: maiden, mother and crone. I was pleased to see a symbol I have been drawn to and using for many years. The representative archetype, the Universal story, such a powerful impression upon the subconscious, was now emblazoned across my mind.

Before I could completely grasp the significance of the message, the scene changed and several of my current clients appeared, one by one, and were enfolded by the glowing angels, snuggly into exquisite wraps. The Divine Mother then came toward me and I could see she held a spirit baby within her loving arms. The archangel Gabriel came forth and presented her with a tiny version of the eloquent blankets; the Divine Mother expertly swathed the baby. She approached one client and sewed the baby neatly and efficiently into the woman's ethereal womb. The Divine Mother repeated this with my other clients, having a spirit baby (or sometimes two) for each one.

I recognized the power of the ritual, and I knew the significance of the gift each woman had received in having the Divine Mother herself bridge the worlds for them—connecting solid and spirit—healing their fertility. They would still have to do their work, of course, and the work is different for each one. Some were further along than others at the time this took place, which was less than two months ago.

Chapter 30

ANGELS & BABIES

"An angel can illuminate the thought and mind of man by strengthening the power of vision."

—*St. Thomas Aquinas*

I have a deck of Archangel Oracle cards by Doreen Virtue. I have taken to shuffling the cards during phone conversations with clients and sometimes, if I am guided to, I bring the cards into the office to see if those clients would like to experience them. One of the archangels is Gabriel. She is female in this particular deck and in some artistic expressions of her. Gabriel—who announced the coming of Jesus to the Virgin Mother—is male in the bible and in some other writings or artwork. It doesn't matter as angels are androgynous anyway. Gabriel is probably feminized often because she is the angel of conception, birth, and beyond, as well as the messenger angel, the angel of writers, journalists, etc.

Talking with a client one day she asked if she was pregnant and I pulled a card from the deck. It was Gabriel, a card called *Nurture* which shows the archangel and others surrounding a sleeping infant. I always take this card to mean yes. That particular client is now pregnant with a baby girl. Another card I find to mean success or yes regarding pregnancy is from the same Archangel deck: *Victory!* The Archangel cards are beautiful and inspirational and I find them to be quite complementary to my spirit baby work.

Angels love spirit baby work and the spirit babies love the angels too. Angels cannot ever help you if you don't ask them to—with the exception of life or death instances that occur before your time—though they desire to do so. I wear a clear quartz crystal angel necklace and have various angel paraphernalia around my home and office. I always call the angels to be with me and thank them for being with me throughout the day and night. I ask for their blessings and inspiration during all client sessions.

One day quite recently I was seated in meditation about an hour before I had a phone session scheduled. The angels were there with me though I didn't have the cards at that moment. A spirit baby appeared before me and I asked him to come to me; I held my hands as I would hold a newborn baby. There he was in my hands, warm and glowing with gold light, and bigger than when I had seen him before. I told him that his mommy was waiting and sent him off, gently, like one would release a butterfly. I reported the experience to his mother a little later during our session.

The angels are amazing and all are dedicated to helping us along our paths. Gabriel, however, seems to be the fertility archangel and she shows up in my life in mysterious ways. One of my clients brought me a wonderful Gabriel candle that is charged with herbs and oils. It smells incredible and I keep it in my office to share the energy with my other clients. I also received a book about Gabriel that has a great deal of information that I had not before known. This supplements the other angel books and cards I have had, some for more than twenty years.

A psychic medium turned out to be in attendance at one of my HypnoFertility® trainings about a year ago. She asked me during a break if I would mind if she told me something, she said she didn't usually do readings when she was the one attending the training but there was something she needed to tell me. I had never met or heard of this woman before she turned up at my class; I said sure. In short, she told me that two guides in particular were working with me: Quan Yin and Gabriel. I had been working with both but nobody knew that because I hadn't mentioned it to anyone. I loved what this lady said because I always get a kick out of such messages.

A client of mine who has been researching Gabriel quite extensively reported that in the bible she'd found the story about Gabriel announcing the impending birth of John the Baptist. The father of John the Baptist apparently argued with Gabriel, citing that he and his wife were too old to have children. Gabriel told the man that a child was definitely to come to him and his wife, that it was God's will. The man continued to argue with the archangel so apparently Gabriel struck him dumb until the child was born.

We must remember that the symbolic content of myth, including Christian myth, according to esteemed Jungian psychologist Dr. Marion Woodman (speaking here mythologically, rather than religiously), is rooted in the human psyche (1985). Mythically, Mary (different from earlier Greek maidens) was immaculately conceived from the womb of Anne. A mature woman who feared she was too old to have a baby Anne meditated and received a visit from an angel. Anne promised the angel: "As the Lord my God liveth, if I bring forth either male or female, I will bring it for a gift unto the Lord my God, and it shall be ministering unto him all the days of its life" (Woodman, 1985, p. 81). In that tradition, like the Divine Child, is the soul child of the spirit.

I love these stories because often one of the issues my clients have is their age. They may have been told they have reduced ovarian reserve, old eggs, that they are too old for one reason or another. Not according to Gabriel! These hopeful examples are very hypnotic and make a powerful impression upon the subconscious mind. There are prayers available to Gabriel that are designed to help with conception, birthing, even adoption. I often work Gabriel prayers into client sessions when requested—combining hypnosis with prayer is awesome. Prayer is said to be the way we talk to God, while hypnosis (meditation) is how God talks to us. This method covers all the bases.

I was pleased to find that neurologist and author Dr. Jill Bolte Taylor uses Angel Cards® several times each day to keep her focused on what she believes to be important in life (2006). Taylor wrote a book called *My Stroke of Insight* which is a fascinating account of the left brain stroke she had a few years ago. She is able to speak from both sides: as a brain scientist and as a patient. This woman's journey is astounding and she effectively identifies right brain/left brain tendencies, as well as energetic effects on healing. Taylor says that her Angel Cards® are one of the most simple and effective tools to help her shift her mind out of the left hemisphere's judgment whenever necessary (Taylor, 2006).

Chapter 31

TO BE OR NOT TO BE?

"Thoughts are just what is. They appear. They're innocent.
They're not personal.
They're like the breeze or the leaves on the trees or the raindrops falling.
Thoughts arise like that, and we can make friends with them.
Would you argue with a raindrop?"

—*Byron Katie*

A woman from Canada called my office some time ago to get some information. She had undergone a great deal of fertility treatment there, and had graduated to coming to a Denver area clinic as many people do. She initially called the office and the HF process was explained to her. She called and e-mailed both my assistants several times but didn't set an appointment even though she told them she was in a time crunch. Eventually we had all spoken to her several times.

When we hadn't heard back from her after a few months I told both Molly and Martie to just forget her and not spend any more time with her if she called back. We are happy to answer questions but in comparing notes the three of us noticed the exact same questions and the exact same verbiage repeatedly. It just seemed odd. A few months later the woman called out of the blue and said she was desperate to get an appointment because this was her last chance and she was about to fly to Denver for her final frozen transfer.

She already knew from her earlier contact with us that this late in the process is not the most ideal time to get started; however, we feel that some hypnosis is better than none in some cases. She begged my assistant for an appointment and agreed to do the recommended minimum of four sessions within the immediate IVF timeframe, and that included the crucial between-transfer-and-pregnancy-test appointment. I was on my way out of town and Molly squeezed her into the one slot I had available before I left and the first one she could get her into upon my return.

I got an unusual vibe from this woman but I decided to see what would unfold—mainly because she was from my hometown. Her behavior was incongruent to her cause and we all could see it; her words didn't match her behavior. But that can happen in the therapy world and is sometimes even the catalyst to healing. On the other hand, my husband and I teach our students that there are only three necessities for successful work with clients—but you've *got* to have them: first, the person must want to be hypnotized/desire the change; second, the person must follow instructions (cooperate); and third, the person must have an IQ above 70. In this case the second point seemed particularly dubious.

I did the first session with this client—she was late for the call. On the second session she called to see if we still had a session booked though the office had confirmed it the day before. As a professional, when I have an appointment booked on my schedule it is set in stone unless I hear or say otherwise; I would assume the same for all professionals. She cancelled the third session, rescheduled, and then when we connected she said that she wondered if she needed the appointment since she was doing so well. Every signal was there with this woman, had been since she first called the office. I include this story here as she has a powerful lesson to teach.

This woman contacted me, so I know that her baby orchestrated the meeting. I could sense her baby but she was not hearing him and she wasn't listening to me either.

Regardless of how much she said she wanted a baby, her behavior said otherwise. She didn't follow instructions or she did so haphazardly. I knew it was game over when she cancelled the session between her transfer and the pregnancy test—that truly is the most critical one. She said she was happy, she was positive, she was fine.

But she hadn't done the work. She hadn't made it her priority and because of that I absolutely knew the IVF would fail. She did have a baby waiting but she wasn't willing to open to the necessary level. That is for her to work out for herself. It does sometimes happen that the mother is not ready for the baby. Sometimes that will shift; sometimes not, as in this case.

Sporadic behavior is a red flag and something everyone at my office pays attention to. At the same time, to see someone transcend their issues is an unparalleled gift and something we all hope will occur. Almost without exception, our client contact is coordinated by the spirit babies. In this case, the baby's presence was strong but the mother couldn't or wouldn't step up to meet it. I believe she has a lot of work to do that she's just not ready for. Everything is as it should be.

Chapter 32

MESSAGES FROM THE SPIRIT BABIES

"It's essential that we understand that taking care of the planet
will be done as we take care of ourselves.
You know that you can't really make much of a difference in things until
you change yourself."

—*Alice Walker*

A 38-year-old acupuncturist came to see me earlier this year. She is also a medical doctor though her license is from a country in Europe so she does not practice medicine here in the United States. She cannot *not* have the knowledge, however, and she had a debilitating fear of Downs Syndrome from her medical school statistics. To protect her privacy we will call her Lucy for the purposes of this writing. Lucy told me that the sum of all of her Western and Eastern medicine knowledge told her that my work was the last piece to her puzzle, and she wanted to do the work so she could have the baby she knew was waiting in the wings.

Lucy was already on her way to becoming healthier on all levels. She was certainly practicing what she preaches in regard to diet, exercise, acupuncture and herbs, and stress reduction. But she also knew that she had some blocks that she needed my help with and she was more than willing to participate in her process. Lucy had suffered three miscarriages and felt she just couldn't get the baby to "stick." She was right in that the issue she was repeatedly experiencing can very well be a response to a subconscious block or emotional trauma.

I worked with Lucy initially to build a foundation upon which to do the deeper work she needed. Her intake uncovered a number of difficulties and stresses she was trying to cope with. For one, her mother lived thousands of miles away and was very ill. Anything involving the mother—subconscious or otherwise—is going to weigh in with this type of work. Being a medical doctor wasn't helping her because she could only draw negatives from her training and her goal was to be positive. She was serious about her healing though and we plunged right in.

One technique I use with clients is to have them talk to an either miscarried or aborted baby(s). I have come to call this my *Rapid Conception Technique* because when I conduct it at the appropriate time in a person's HF it tends to result in a somewhat sooner-than-later healthy pregnancy—in just the right time and in just the right way, of course. I have a unique way of carrying out this process and I have yet to even teach my technique to others. I will actually be including it for the first time as part of my revised and updated HypnoFertility® training in August 2013 at the National Guild of Hypnotists' Summer Institute in Marlborough, MA.

I'm going to skip straight to Lucy's experience with her babies that day in my office not long after I had met her. We started with the usual intake/update and then she curled up in the burgundy beanbag (metaphorical womb) and we began the hypnotic process. Lucy rapidly drifted into a deep state of hypnosis yet also remained aware of my presence and was able to communicate with me through ideomotor response (finger signals) and verbally when necessary. This way I could monitor and facilitate her experience and as it unfolded she could participate interactively if she so desired while also absorbing the benefits of profound hypnotic peace.

Lucy's babies appeared to her almost immediately and she was able to interact with each one. She reported later that they had given her great insight and that she was surprised that they'd been so "friendly and easy." The babies told her that she had done a good job reconciling her childhood and then one baby came forward and told Lucy that she must heal her biggest wound. The baby didn't specify exactly what that was but did indicate that the healing would shift the alignment and her babies would then begin to enter—to be born into the physical world to share her and her husband's journey of life.

Lucy was ecstatic and she knew that she would heal that wound simply by continuing with the process she and I had begun. We followed what was unfolding in her life—whatever her psyche purged we addressed as needed. Less than three months after Lucy experienced my *Rapid Conception Technique* she was naturally pregnant. She is excitedly awaiting the birth of her first child, and she knows there are more to follow. The babies made that abundantly clear during the session, and I could see multiple spirit baby lights buzzing around Lucy during our sessions.

I utilize this process quite often with clients so I have lots of examples to choose from. I'm going to include two of my favorites here for your benefit—so you can share in the knowledge that comes from direct contact with your spirit baby. This client was a Skype client from another state. We had done a good deal of work together when she flew out to Denver to meet with me in person. Samantha is a 44-year-old research scientist who spent a great deal of time earning her PhD and working her way up the ranks of her field. She and her husband are both originally from overseas (different places) so their families are scattered virtually across the planet.

Samantha too snuggled into the beanbag, covered with soft blankets of lavender and pink. I hypnotized her, then guided her on a beautiful journey through healing waters and sacred mists and even variations of time. A baby boy appeared to her and her face lit up with joy. He told her she was right on track (she had an IVF cycle coming up soon). Samantha then noticed what she called a snuggly, playful spirit baby over to her left. Then one appeared directly in front of her face that seemed to have stronger energy, she felt; perhaps this one would be coming first.

Samantha reported that the babies were putting things in front of her, showing her that she needed to get back to what she called her Mother Mary stuff. The babies let Samantha know that they were aware of the things she was doing and advised her to erase old stuff, and to follow her gut. Samantha was excited to have this encounter with her babies and she played with them and just resonated with their energies. She then reported that there were "other spirit babies here."

A baby with an orange/coppery aura told her that time is shifting, times have changed. Special souls are incarnating and it is really important for that shift. The baby said there are a lot of souls with the colors of indigo and green, and that there are changes needed. A shift, a growth in the mothers is what is needed to prepare them for their parts in this; the fertility path is a realignment. Samantha said the orange/coppery spirit baby told her that she had diverted from her spiritual path but her fertility journey had realigned her. (Archangel Gabriel's aura is copper.)

Feeling and seeing purple now, Samantha reported that Walter (Makichen) had popped into her mind. She spoke directly to me and said that "he is here, he comes here, he is with you." Walter then told her she is definitely going to have a baby. Samantha reported what she called a really strong vibration on her left side; she then identified it as Walter telling her to follow her spiritual path. He told my client (during her experience) that he is still very involved, and still doing this work. He was surrounded by spirit babies and he and they told Samantha that they brought her to me, and that the best possible preparation for IVF is hypnosis, meditation, writing, and yoga.

I found this session with Samantha particularly interesting because it seemed to have a strong resemblance to the experience I mentioned earlier when the spirit babies appeared to my client, Teri. And Samantha isn't the first client I've had who has had Walter show up. One client I had reported nearly verbatim what Samantha said, including the part about Walter. This client, Mary, is a 46-year-old woman who has done deep work to connect with her femininity—her Divine Feminine. She has elected to conceive naturally while intricately pursuing her spirituality.

Mary, too, has connected with her spirit baby, and has seen all the little spirit baby lights flying around my office. She has also received messages from them, and Walter has shown up in more than one of her sessions to assure her that she will have her baby. I am amazed at just how many people have independently encountered the spirit babies in my office, and reported nearly identical experiences. Walter confirms that the act of simply connecting with a spirit baby and feeling its presence can help prospective parents to overcome their worries and fears (Makichen, 2005). Students from our various trainings, clients; even a dog witnessed this phenomenon.

I had the pleasure this summer of conducting a private training for a lovely woman who had done the hypnotherapy certification training with us during the spring. I enjoy the one-on-one trainings because I am able to personalize them and the student can spend more or less time on various topics as it best suits her. I believe in learning by doing; I don't think you can learn this work well if you have nothing but theory, therefore I incorporate hypnosis into both my group classes and my private ones. However, during a private training the student is able to experience actual sessions just as the client would; in group I can only manage generalized group experiences.

My student wanted to meet the spirit babies so that was the focus of a session I did with her on the second day of training. Ingrid snuggled into the beanbag chair just as so many women had done before her. I hypnotized her and took her into a deep, nourishing state. I cleared any potential blocks or psychic debris, balanced her mind, body, and spirit, and then had her energetically bathe in crystal clear divine light. From a state of pure peace Ingrid silently welcomed any contact from the spirit babies.

Within seconds a brilliant smile spread across Ingrid's face—a big, golden baby (as she described it) had appeared before her. The golden spirit baby affirmed her purpose in the HF process and Ingrid was elated. She too was enlightened as to the needs of the spirit babies: aligning the energies; shifting vibrations; their mothers' life purpose/spiritual adjustments; the need for sensitive, educated, well-placed souls to soothe and heal the Earth Mother; and all that had been revealed to me, to my clients, and to those I have mentioned throughout this book. Sparkly little spirit baby orbs flitted around the room while Ingrid dialogued with the golden baby; the energy in the room was incredible.

The golden spirit baby shared with Ingrid a glimpse of her path and affirmed that she was exactly on track. She could barely sit still after the session, she was so excited. We did manage to complete the training and within weeks we received word from Ingrid that she had found an unbelievable office space opportunity. Shortly thereafter she let us know that she had booked her first HypnoFertility® client and that things were coming together better than she had even thought possible. Since then Ingrid is happily carrying on, pursuing her dreams and assisting spirit babies and their parents.

Now, that dog I mentioned. One of our hypnotherapy graduates now works as a training assistant for our school. She was at the office one day, down on the lower level, involved in some kind of organizing task; she had brought her handsome, furry, red dog Cena with her and he was downstairs too. I had just seen three HF clients in a row and had another one due in a few minutes. I knew Cena pretty well as Holly often brought him to the school with her.

I wanted to say a quick hello to them so I headed downstairs and entered the lower level office. Cena just stared and stared at me and wouldn't budge—usually he comes right over to me—then he just sat down. He plopped his rear end right to the floor while the front half of him continued to stare at me, his eyes wandering somewhat around my head. Holly exclaimed that she had never seen him like that, that she had no idea what was wrong with him. I laughed and said, "Oh it must be the spirit babies, they hang out in my aura and I've been working with a lot of their mothers today."

Cena apparently got used to the sparkly babes and finally came over to greet me—albeit cautiously. I chatted with him and Holly for a few minutes before heading back up to my office. I saw Holly a few weeks later and she told me that before she met Drake and took this amazing hypnotherapy journey, she never would have believed such a thing. She was still amazed that she had taken my spirit baby explanation without so much as blinking; had not only accepted it, but actually believed it to be true. Cena's reaction had basically floored her, but Holly was able to integrate the experience and access the next level of her own spiritual growth. Kind of a fun example but at the same time you can see the spirit babies doing their cherished work, making their presence known, and helping someone to learn and grow spiritually and on all levels.

Chapter 33

THE BETWEEN BY PROXY

"Love is the only way to grasp another human being in the innermost core of his personality."

— *Victor Frankel*

Having experienced the spirit babies during my own life purpose regression, and having encountered them through my client, Teri, and then again during other client and even student sessions, I decided to see if I—while at the helm—could send someone there for the express purpose of dialogue and understanding. Our office assistant, Martie, has meditated and practiced yoga for more than three decades, and she has also taken our training, and worked with private hypnotherapy clients. I asked her if she would be willing to be hypnotized for the purpose of entering *The Between* and investigating the *Spirit Baby Whisperer* energies. She said yes. Following is the transcript of the session (after the initial hypnosis and Martie having entered *The Between*; she is responding to the question of what the spirit babies would like us to know):

Deep, deep in the center of my mind, feel at home here. Beings— life is all one, not individual babies. One living mind, pure mind, pure spirit, given thoughts that are transmuted into words, comes to me as a wholeness, completeness, finding words to describe it. Communion. Essence of life = spirit/mind. What is born in form is not an individual but a part of all being, all mind.

Let it come forth knowing itself—not anonymous, not separate. Let me come forth knowing myself; that I can lead others to peace. I am one but appear to be many, but still I am one. Let me come forth knowing myself. I will appear to be many but I am one.

Ease the vessel, the mother, into a unified state. Integrate, harmonize, balance, unite. I shall appear to be many—I am one—will come forth as one, knowing myself, and deliver peace. Ease the vessel, the mother, into unity. Potentialities, prospects, possibilities . . . If she's eased and integrated I can come forth.

There's potential. No time, it's always now. Forever now, always now. Truth, not all, all can, all could bring forth, only some can be eased into unity that I who appear to be many come forth knowing myself. (The babies, Spirit, speaking through Martie; I asked for a name. The name I received was) **Beloved.**

Understand it isn't the mechanical act of bringing forth that matters, it's the bringing forth in unity and oneness; otherwise what is brought forth is lost in fragments. Ease the vessel into unity that I may come forth as one knowing myself.

(I ask for input on the difficulty some women have conceiving as compared to others.) Some have babies easily; some so much struggle. Is there a reason? Yes and no. Mechanical level. Conceiving is a mechanical act; some conceive more easily. Bringing forth is a spiritual act, an act of sharing; a different level. The vessel, the mother, can conceive in disunity but will bring forth only in unity. Said set aside for special purpose. Love creates.

What is the purpose for desiring conception? Love, there are motives for conceiving that are not love. Where there is love it's easy. Where love is the motive, bringing forth is easy, natural. Ease them into unity with love. There isn't always a superficial answer (Beloved's response to my question of how easily crack addicts and such have babies— something my clients always want to know). Put them in contact with their true self inwardly and they'll know if they love or if they want for something other than love to make them whole—show them their wholeness. Let them see their love, take them in (hypnosis), where it is, deep, deep, deep, deep, show them the light within each one. Help them to see their innocence (direction to me), to know that they're worthy to bring forth. Some don't believe that secretly; the secret is that they don't believe they're worthy to bring forth. Show them innocence, purity, worthiness; show them the light.

(Beloved is coming to the end of transmission, addresses the Spirit Baby Whisperer process once again.) It's occurring now, always, forever, now. Your motive must be love as well (addressing my ability to resonate with my clients—same frequency). Your own innocence is clear to you. Remember, the giver receives. The receiver gives. It's all one.

Chapter 34

TV: SEEING THE LIGHT?

"We are still masters of our fate. We are still captains of our souls."

—*Winston Churchill*

The need to apply hypnotherapy techniques to infertility situations is essential. Women have been subjected to so much trauma during this journey that their own bodies turn against them, making natural or medically assisted conception close to impossible. Invasive medical procedures and feeling like you are not being heard or that you are a number rather than a human being is painful. The more this occurs, the more it compounds, and the worse you feel.

The very second you walk into some clinics they sit you down to crunch numbers and run an immediate credit check on you. Others insist that you have a mammogram before they will work with you. This just adds to the turmoil you're already experiencing—it's a domino effect: one hits another, and then another; only with these dominoes each one that tips is causing fear; emotional, physical, and/or financial stress; worry; self-deprecation; sometimes relationship strain; and much more.

As I've said, compounding is a form of hypnosis and the stronger the emotion attached the stronger the reinforcement. Compounding can come from health care or complementary care practitioners, statistics, the internet, friends or family, television, and many other experiences. Not too terribly long ago some of my clients were watching a certain celebrity broadcasting her fertility journey on television for the world to see. As I have said many times, the subconscious does not differentiate between what is real and what is imagination (or fantasy or pretend or make-believe). That includes television.

I'm sure most of you are familiar with the case as it is part of a reality show: basically, the woman was required to do a mammogram, was diagnosed with breast cancer, and ended up with a double mastectomy rather than the baby she desired. This TV star and her husband did eventually utilize the services of a gestational carrier to become the parents of a baby boy. While I am glad to hear they had a happy ending, I'm less than impressed that the whole story was not only aired on a TV show, but also picked up by the various news media—not to mention the tabloids—and kept in the public eye for a great deal of time.

This case only compounded the fears of everyday fertility clients who are just trying to keep it together. Mammogram testing should be a private, personal experience; as should any fertility issues and related decisions be. We have to remember that television amplifies issues for the purpose of entertainment. That includes so-called reality shows as well as sit coms or dramas or whatever else you might be drawn to watch. Several police officers and detectives I know have told me the same thing: if everyone on the planet was murdered at the rate they are on television, there would simply be no one left at all.

We also must remember that it takes a certain personality type to take on any given job. Someone drawn to becoming a reality star may have a personality or mood disorder, show narcissistic or histrionic tendencies—in other words need to be the center of attention or be a "drama queen." Not everyone is the same but in the psychology field we do sometimes see such propensities. On the other hand, I have worked with several Hollywood actresses, writers, and producers. You don't know who they are because they don't want you to—their fertility issues are something they desire to keep quiet.

Their secrets are safe with me, of course, because all my sessions are confidential. Ethically, confidentiality must be kept; and it's also the law. I would never breech anyone's confidence, but the point here is that if those Hollywood clients had just wanted to get attention, they would have revealed their crises. Instead, they took comfort in being able to get the assistance they needed from me, and were grateful to keep it quiet just as I have recommended in *It's Conceivable!*, and in virtually every fertility related thing I do or say.

When Prince William married Princess Kate, I told my husband and several colleagues to *watch and see how fast she has "infertility."* She's only 27-years-old so it would be pretty unusual for her to have any difficulty—as princesses go, anyway. Then again, infertility is the hot topic of the moment. There were a few statements about possible infertility directly following the wedding, but as of a few weeks ago multiple tabloids had front page stories to the effect of *Kate begins infertility treatments.* Once she was pregnant they couldn't wait to publicize hospitalization for NVP or morning sickness, and we shouldn't expect things to change as the pregnancy progresses.

All in all I hope this chapter puts television and tabloid—and overall celebrity hyperbole—into perspective. When you are subjected to such information, please consider the likelihood of amplification and adjust your own responses accordingly. Utilize your tools, particularly the simple but powerful *cancel technique* and use your hypnosis to maintain balance. Focus on your spirit baby and keep in mind the 3 keys: meditate, listen, trust.

Chapter 35

PINK CANDLES

*"What the caterpillar calls the end of the world,
the master calls a butterfly."*

— *Richard Bach*

I had a phone client a few years ago who was undergoing IVF. We had been working together for a couple of months and in that time she and her husband had accumulated several healthy frozen embryos. The clinic was ready to transfer two of the embryos but neither my client nor her husband wanted boys. They were privy to gender and able to request two female embryos to be transferred. My client told me they wanted twins: two girls.

As I have said I have no direct control over such things but I will reinforce the desire during the hypnotic process—it never hurts to ask. As I prepared to record this client's session, I was guided to light two small pink candles. I did so and then proceeded to create the recording. When I am in session I find myself in a trancelike state, focused on my client and her specifics, intuition at the helm. In hypnotism this is called uptime trance. The client—who does not need to make any conscious effort whatsoever during her session—is in what we call downtime trance.

I had forgotten all about the candles until the conclusion of the recording, at which time I looked over at them and discovered one had burned all the way down while the other had stopped burning very early on. I knew immediately that this meant my client would have one baby this time. One healthy girl.

I did not tell my client this information because from a hypnotic standpoint it is not going to be helpful to her. A few weeks later my client knew for sure: there was one baby girl. I congratulated her and reminded her that everything unfolds exactly as it needs to. We can never know the reasons, but perhaps my client would have been unable to carry twins, or perhaps the child she was carrying needed to come in alone. We can speculate endlessly, but this is where we must trust the Universe. My client was, of course, elated to have her healthy baby daughter.

Chapter 36

RESOLVING MOTHER

"The moment a child is born, the mother is also born. She never existed before. The woman existed, but the mother, never. A mother is something absolutely new."

—*Rajneesh*

Mother issues are incredibly prominent with my clients. That is not to say that everyone has them or that they are a catch-all analysis. It does make sense, of course, that relationship (or lack thereof) with Mother would contribute to fertility, pregnancy and birthing difficulties. We do feel our mothers' feelings in utero and we are doused with stressor hormones anytime she is (on the plus side that goes for endorphins too). We are connected nervous system to nervous system for 40 weeks. And then we grow up with her. Separation from Mother, whether by death, due to illness, or because she is emotionally unavailable, has its own difficulties. Resolving Mother issues is often the key to conception, it is in and of itself a subconscious release, and it alleviates the fears of being the same kind of mother or—in something less understood by the general population but incredibly familiar to therapists—not being as good a mother as one's mother, not being able to measure up.

According to author and trauma psychologist Alice Miller (1997), it is quite apparent sometimes that people could not possibly have survived the sheer amount of pain that accompanied them through childhood. In such cases, they repress their feelings. If a woman has to repress her needs because of her own mother, they will surface from deep within the psyche and attempt to gratify themselves through her own child—regardless of how educated she may be, or how much she may think she can stop it. And even though a person may be consciously aware of, or have insight into, any given trauma, Dr. Woodman reiterates that if it is not released subconsciously it will most definitely continue to resurface (Woodman, 1985).

As to the psyche, for as long as we are in and of this world, says Woodman (1985), the psyche is enacted—that is to say, expressed—through the medium of the body. The soul, of course, is a great deal more than the "portion" of the body itself. The soul is not limited to manifesting in the physical body alone; the soul manifests in what we consider to be the infinite body that constitutes the so-called "body" of the imagination, and which includes the entire world of the visionary arts: music, dance, poetry, sculpture, painting, etc.

Denial or repression of childhood trauma is destructive. It's not that you have to confront anyone; but if you don't acknowledge your own issues they will manifest as symptoms in the body. If they are mother related, in particular, you will eventually have no choice but to address them. Regarding the psyche, or subconscious mind, Woodman (1985) has findings similar to mine, to Dr. Miller's, and to Dr. Herman's as cited throughout this writing. Any wounding in the body, says Woodman (1985), will produce a tremendous release of healing energy at the point of the blockage. The goal of energy healing methods designed for individuals with such issues is to identify what the soul is trying to do, then relax the body so the soul can do it.

In *Drama of the Gifted Child* author Alice Miller (1997) states:

One such consequence is the person's inability to experience consciously certain feelings . . . either in childhood or later in adulthood . . . These people have all developed the art of not experiencing feelings, for a child can experience her feelings only when there is somebody there who accepts her fully, understands her, and supports her. If that person is missing, if the child must risk losing the mother's love or the love of her substitute in order to feel, then she will repress her emotions. She cannot even experience them secretly, "just for herself;" she will fail to experience them at all. But they will nevertheless stay in her body, in her cells, stored up as information that can be triggered by a later event.

Because these events can and do take up residence in a woman's body, it is essential that they be addressed. Denial and other defense mechanisms may fool the conscious mind but the subconscious mind is home to the emotions. They can toil and boil and simmer and even cool. But they are there nonetheless and they *will* express themselves. In fact, they *are* expressing themselves; you just may or may not recognize it. Intellectualization is a common defense mechanism of women from abusive backgrounds. Intellectualization holds great power, however, as Miller (1997) confirms: if the mind ignores the vital messages of the body, the results can be disastrous.

"Blaming the mother" has virtually become cliché. But we are not looking to blame anyone—only to release subconscious blocks that may well be impeding your fertility— so please bear with me a little longer. That said, it is perhaps a gift from the subconscious mind to block fertility until you are able to identify and then process any childhood residue, regardless of how it came to be. This does not have to take a long time. I am certainly a supporter of more traditional methods of counseling or therapy and I recommend them to people quite regularly. I also recognize, however, that people often find talk therapy a long road to follow and are frightened—rightly so in many cases—that they won't make their healing destination in time.

You must start from wherever you are and not having spent time in therapy is not detrimental to your success. Initiating the process is like shining a bright light into a dark corner: shadows dissolve. In so doing you are making a declaration to the psyche and giving yourself permission to embrace your own healing and align your energy with your baby's. So, if you feel you'd like to undertake something like psychoanalysis, but are concerned with your biological clock, know that you can receive great benefit from it as you continue your HypnoFertility® and as far beyond as you desire to continue. Hypnosis, as I said earlier, is considered *rapid change* therapy, and though we may work together for twelve weeks (give or take) I can often clear the mother issues in a session or two.

One woman I saw a few years ago had been turned down for IVF by one of the local clinics. They had performed surgery on her during which a surgical instrument had become imbedded in her uterus. A second surgery was done to remove it but they were unable to get the whole thing. They didn't want to compromise her uterus any further by making another attempt and they told her they would not accept her as an IVF patient. Devastated, the woman found me and came in as soon as she could get an appointment.

Talking with her I got the strongest sense that this was all something to do with her mother. I inquired and she agreed: her mother had given birth to her at a young age (around 18) as a result of an unplanned pregnancy. This indicated that my client was an unwanted child which she confirmed. She was parenting her parents and two younger siblings. She had also chosen to work in a helping profession in which she was witness to results of trauma in many children.

I conducted a clearing session on both of these powerful issues. Immediately feeling relief and release, my client said she was filled with hope once again. We continued working together for a while and within two cycles she was naturally pregnant. We worked throughout the pregnancy, in particular to support her uterus. She gave birth to a healthy baby boy despite the fact that her reproductive endocrinologist had deemed it impossible.

Dr. Marion Woodman (1985) author of *The Pregnant Virgin—a Process of Psychological Transformation* writes:

The puella *mother who has never taken up residence in her own body, and therefore fears her own chthonic nature, is not going to experience pregnancy as a quiet meditation with her unborn child, nor birth as a joyful bonding experience. Although she may go through the motions of natural childbirth, the psyche/soma split in her is so deep that physical bonding between her and her baby daughter does not take place. Her child lives with a profound sense of despair, a despair which becomes conscious if in later years she does active imagination with her body and releases waves of grief and terror that resonate with the initial, primal rejection.*

Dr. Woodman puts the absolute necessity of what I like to call "doing your own work" quite succinctly. The above quote reinforces the importance of the releasing process described in Chapter 2. Balance of mind, body, and spirit must be created and maintained, and subconscious blocks must be acknowledged and cleared, not only to heal fertility, but to support a healthy pregnancy, a peaceful birth, and secure attachment for the child.

Clients may recognize themselves in the puella mother referenced by Woodman (1985) above. The insightful paragraph may also illustrate the needs of the inner child— acknowledged, perhaps, for the first time. As might Alice, through the looking glass, recognize the truth; penetrate the surface though she knows it's upside down. In other words, no matter how painful, no matter how confusing—whether it is you as a mother, or you as a child, or your own mother, however you relate to the statement—you can heal from distorted truths, overcome false surfaces.

This type of issue will not go away no matter how long you ignore it or resist it. But on the bright side you know that techniques are available to help you release, reframe, integrate the experience as appropriate. In so doing you clear your energy, your life heals in ways you may never have imagined, and you align with your baby's energy. In this kind of releasing work you are breaking a cycle; on many levels healing energy freely flows.

Chapter 57

LONGING FOR A BABY

"When a woman conceives her true self, a miracle occurs and life around her begins again."

—*Marianne Williamson*

I would like to address here that my practice is all inclusive and accepting. I do not judge my clients regardless of what they are, think, feel, or fear. I have single clients in my practice: women who are single but becoming pregnant by choice. This is done in many ways; I just ascertain the whens, whys, and hows, and support them accordingly. Age, IVF, donor sperm related procedures, IVF donor sperm/donor egg, adopted embryos, borrowing a male friend certain days of the cycle . . . again, whatever your circumstance, however you choose to proceed, I will support you in every way.

Lesbian clients have similar issues to single women (as far as sperm acquisition) though they do, of course, (usually) have a partner. Again, the route the two of you have elected to take—in other words the details—is totally your business and I will support you across the board. Every client is different, every relationship is different, yet at the same time there are some common elements that crop up simply because you are women. The methods I utilize to help so-called traditional couples (one man/one woman) are applicable to everyone with an occasional tweaking depending on the context.

Some gay men desire to be parents also. They are the most limited because without a uterus having a child is a creative endeavor. A gestational carrier is one option for men but it can be a very expensive process. Having a female friend carry the child is another option, however if she is to go through the medical method of being inseminated there will be a lot of tests and details. I can help the couple with stress in enduring the sometimes quite lengthy process; I can also work with the surrogate to receive the sperm, the embryos, etc. and just support the entire experience.

Sometimes there is an issue with HIV and even though everyone may be consciously fine with it, there can be subconscious blocks that impede the procedure all along the way. In these cases I can clear any blockages and get things back on track. I can do a lot with bonding also so you can certainly bring the baby in and we can all work together. I can help with stress, with choices you might need to make; I can support adoption if that's what you'd like to do. Hypnotic bonding and what we call reparenting is extremely powerful for adopted babies/children (adults too for that matter).

I always inquire as to specific religious preferences and I will ask for your input and direction and work it into the sessions accordingly. Prayers are powerful when given at the deepest level of mind and I will include any prayers you might desire. Practicing Catholic women, for example, do not do IVF. Beyond that, for IUI their husband's sperm must be gathered in a special condom during intercourse and brought to the clinic for the insemination process. Not all Catholics practice by these rules.

I could elaborate quite a bit here but the purpose of this chapter is to let you know that whatever your personal circumstances or choices or needs, etc. you are welcome in my practice. I can help you; HF therapists can help you. You are cared about and supported—there is no judgment. At this point I realize that you've read quite a bit about the spirit babies so I'll just give you a brief reminder that they are choosing you. They want and need your specific circumstances to fulfill their life purposes—they can't wait to be with you.

Chapter 38

CASE STUDIES

*So often times it happens that we live our lives in chains
and we never even know we have the key.*

—*The Eagles*

Women struggling with infertility often call or e-mail my office with questions or looking for information. In many ways this is the reason I've written this book—to help you to better understand the work I do. I am including here some brief case studies; my intention is that you can get an idea of what some of my clients present with, their ages, careers, diagnoses, procedures, number of sessions or timeframe, pregnancy, etc. These are real clients; I haven't included every detail in their files—the highlights are most important here.

Some of these clients have had abortions; some have survived abusive childhoods or other traumas. I included them where (and if) appropriate. I didn't specify exactly what tools or protocols were utilized—I include most everything I've described throughout this book, combined with personal contributions from clients, to create my clients' individualized sessions.

Case A

A 49-year-old client had undergone 2 failed IVF donor cycles. She intuitively knew it was the stress that was preventing her success so, having had a positive experience with hypnosis many years before, she decided she needed hypnotherapy and made an appointment with my office.

On session #1 I was aware of strong spirit baby lights (which I noted on my client's file). We did the intake and proceeded to begin our HF work. I was pleased to have a few weeks before the transfer so that I would have enough time to address all that was going on for my client.

Glancing through her file I noticed that on session #2 I saw the baby very close to her right side, and that on session #3 the baby was really close to her head. I had no doubt this baby was coming and that my client's up and coming transfer would be a success. That day I received the word "him" which I noted on her file. On session #4 I received "him" again and saw him to the left of his mother, then hovering over her throat chakra. During her hypnosis session I had her invite her baby into her life and I saw him (in energetic form) fly straight into her arms. This was 2 weeks prior to transfer.

Her fifth session occurred just prior to transfer and her sixth was the crucial waiting period session: between transfer and pregnancy test results. It was at that time that my client told me her baby had come to her in a dream and given her his name: Boone. As I write this Boone's birth is imminent. His EDD is 12/27/2012. His mom said she sailed through her pregnancy and that the doctors couldn't believe how easy things were going for her. She joked that it was almost like they had to make up drama by the end of her pregnancy.

Boone's mother saw me for 12 sessions: 5 pre-transfer, 1 immediately following, the other 6 as needed throughout the pregnancy, and a couple preceding the birth. She plans to come after the baby is born on an as needed basis.

Case B

I worked with a 43-year-old client for 22 sessions over an 18-month timeframe. She'd had several failed IUIs but desperately wanted to conceive naturally. The baby was present with her from the beginning; the process was very much hers to embrace. Eventually. This client did have a lot of emotional difficulties to work through, including mother issues—which she did. She and her husband were very healthy: athletic, vegan, non-believers in drugs of any sort. She stated adamantly that she wanted no meds; that the IUIs had been against her true wishes. I supported her throughout all of this. I knew the baby was there and I had no doubt he would come through in time.

It eventually became apparent to my client that IVF was needed. She was miserable but at that point I utilized HF to help her come to terms with what mattered to her most: her baby. I worked with her to welcome the drugs into her body with love and peace. I sent her to Conceptions because I knew they would treat her kindly and truly respect her feelings, needs, and preferences. My client did conceive IVF donor and once that part of the ordeal was over she was thrilled. Pregnant with her baby boy she happily told me one day that she had come to terms with everything, that her husband was thrilled, and that she was ready to "be in the now" and "enjoy her future with her baby."

Case C

A 36-year-old client came in because she had a highly stressful job where she worked with traumatized children. This is often a major block to fertility because there is so much negative emotion; in this case brutal visuals conveyed through psychological interview and/or through debriefing with other therapists or reading charts. I knew I had my work cut out for me to clear this woman's subconscious blocks. Not surprisingly, she was diagnosed with unexplained infertility. I could see this woman's spirit baby bopping around even as she related her 5 failed IUIs and years of trying to conceive. On the 1st session the baby was above her head and then he moved over to her left elbow. By the 2nd session he was by her right shoulder. She was considering IVF but by the 4th session she was pregnant—"Without even trying," she said gleefully. No need for IVF. She managed to keep the secret and told her partner on his birthday, a couple of weeks after she found out. After a carefree pregnancy and peaceful birth, my client sent me the cutest picture of her new little boy.

Case D

A 39-year-old client did some phone work with me from California. She also was able to come into my office a time or two. By the time I met her she'd had 3 failed IVFs with the 3rd cycle being "devastating" in her words. She'd gotten 11 follicles but only 1 egg. During her 4th round she told me she'd gotten 9 mature eggs but only 1 that was chromosomally normal. Her desire was to get more and then get them to blastocyst for testing. With so many obstacles I knew that to deal with them this woman needed emotional balance and tools.

By her 5th session with me—a phone session—my client was 6½ weeks pregnant. I could feel the baby strongly and I knew all was well with him. My client told me that, "in this journey I have developed faith." We utilized the hypnotic process the rest of her pregnancy, for the birth, and afterward as well. She told me that she'd had a fantastic pregnancy despite what others had tried to tell her.

Case E

A 38-year-old telephone client from the east side of the country called to say it was her "last chance." She'd had 3 failed IVFs and was on her 4th. They had 1 normal day-3 embryo, frozen. I was able to ascertain 2 bright spirit babies on the one occasion she came into the office. I can see/sense them for phone/Skype clients also—it just happened the babies were particularly bright and shiny that day. My client was relocating overseas so there was a lot of stress there along with her IVF woes. She also had some regrets she needed to come to terms with and by diligently doing her work she was able to clear her psyche in those matters.

Not long before she was to move my client transferred her single 8-cell embryo. The doctors told her there was basically no chance. But, as so often happens when HypnoFertility® is used in tandem with other procedures, she conceived. Sometime after her baby girl was born she got in touch to send pictures and to tell us what an excellent pregnancy and birth she had experienced.

Case F

A 40-year-old client came in with low ovarian reserve and high FSH. She belonged to a group called *Single Mothers by Choice*. She had experienced 3 failed IUIs and was thinking about IVF and donor. She was considering the financial costs and told me, "My goal is to be a mom, not to be a mom at any cost with my own eggs." Part of her work was coming to a decision that was absolutely right for her. She did.

On the 4th session I saw a bright baby to the top right of her head. I got "she" as did my client. Having decided to go to another state to do her IVF donor, my client and I worked together throughout the duration of her journey. At one point she needed a laminaria and I did hypnosis specifically for that. Her procedure went very smoothly as happens when hypnosis is utilized for such circumstances. The doctor told her that her cervix was "quite a way up in her body and also on a weird angle."

As a single mom my client had some fears to contend with and we discussed how fear masquerades as intuition. At session #12 I had a very strong sense/vision of a female and on session #13 "his" came in. I wasn't sure at the time if she was transferring 1 or 2 but as it turned out my client elected to transfer 2 embryos. After her positive pregnancy test we shifted our focus to keeping her little twins safe inside. She ended up on bed rest a few weeks before the babies were due so we worked by phone. More quickly than I could have imagined possible my client e-mailed us an announcement and pictures of her baby son and daughter.

Case G

A 43-year-old woman was referred to me by a medical doctor colleague I often cross refer with. This woman had a lot of issues to contend with including high FSH, a previous abortion, and serious issues with her husband around trying to get pregnant. At the same time she wanted to make a significant career change. The intake showed a lot of background work that would need to be addressed in order for this client to process her fertility issues. She jumped in eagerly and we worked together to clear subconscious blocks, to release various traumas, and to explore exactly what the situation was with her husband.

After about a half dozen sessions my client came to a somewhat dizzying conclusion. By that I mean, in following her heart and her intuition, she elected to shake up her life and follow her bliss. She decided to divorce her husband and leave the state to pursue her education and her new career. About a year later my client got in touch with me to let me know she was elated with her choices and living "happily childless."

I include this client's case because it is one of the rare occasions when someone comes in thinking she is pursuing one thing and her path unfolds differently than she expected. I have mentioned before that this is unusual and there are a couple of significant differences between this client and my other clients that we must note: I did not see or sense any spirit babies around this woman as we worked together in my office; she suspected her husband was gay and the assessment of that possibility took precedence over the initial fertility piece. Incidentally, she became an elementary school teacher and interacts with little ones in the way that best suits her—and them—and she, the last time I spoke with her, assured me she is thrilled with the outcome of her process and thanked me immensely for just holding the space and allowing her *to be* so her own unique path could unfold.

Case H

Another recent client is a 43-year-old woman from the Caribbean. I worked with her both by Skype and in person when she flew out to do some work at our clinic for about a week. Initial intake revealed that this woman had experienced 3 IUIs and suffered 3 miscarriages, plus she had experienced 1 failed IVF. Her diagnosis was unexplained infertility. This truly lovely woman had read the book *Spirit Babies* and told me that she always felt she had 2 babies with her. She was concerned that her babies were cross with her because of some of the writings in the book (which I addressed early on).

She had a number of issues to address—it almost feels like paving a road sometimes when you begin the work. My client took her work seriously and dedicated herself to aligning with her little ones. Her spirit babies were often "flying around" (as it appears to me) and I'd see them around her on the computer screen but also in my own office or whatever location I was in. The mother of these sparkly orbs had a lesson to learn before they could come through—patience. I was very aware of this and I reminded her often as well. She embraced the tools I provided as we worked together and though it could, at times, be frustrating for her, she stuck with it and allowed me to provide the support necessary for what was truly becoming an energetic transformation.

I had told my client about my son, Dylan—his proclamation of being the first HF baby, and the insights he had shared with me over the years. Upon arriving in Denver, my client asked if she could meet Dylan. I asked him and he agreed. I brought Dylan in and introduced him to my client. I left them to chat and didn't hear what was said. My client later told me that Dylan had said she would definitely get pregnant. Dylan told me basically the same thing and also mentioned that he felt it would be twins.

This client did 12 sessions with me altogether. A few months after she'd returned to her oceanic paradise we received word that she was 12 weeks pregnant with twins. The babies have not yet been born but their due date is fast approaching.

Case I

A 41-year-old physician conceived and gave birth naturally to a baby son. Prior to the blessed event, this woman had been through a horrible ordeal: having lost one baby from heart problems and one from a chromosome 18 issue at 20 and 14 weeks respectively; dealing with grief; and dealing with high FSH, low ovarian reserve, fertility drugs, failed IUIs and failed IVFs. Her job was busy and stressful and, as is always a danger in the medical world, she had been subjected to a great deal of trauma over the years: injury, death, etc. (As you'll recall, these events create subconscious imprints and can seriously exacerbate infertility, anxiety, and other such issues.) She told me she always felt like she was waiting for the other shoe to drop—understandably so.

Upon learning of this woman's background I was not surprised to find her navigating so much chaos. She had many other issues which I won't go into in detail; she did 12 sessions with me and we worked through them. I met with her at my office once when she was in the Denver area, other than that we met by phone. We cleared a good many subconscious blocks and laid the foundation for a healthy, uneventful pregnancy. After having to cancel yet another IVF cycle for lack of follicles, my client decided to try the donor route. I have a mantra of sorts that I often repeat during my hypnosis sessions and that tends to stick in my clients' minds: my baby is coming in just the right time and in just the right way. It really is the perfect statement to welcome your child because it covers all the options.

My client and her husband had ended up with quite a few healthy donor blasts, but before arrangements could be made to transfer any of them my client discovered that she was naturally pregnant. We worked together to get her past the "critical" points (the times she lost her other babies) and once we were past those our focus was on keeping the little sweetie inside until it was time for his birth. He was born full term—a perfectly healthy little boy with two elated parents.

Case J

This is another baby who snuck right in under IVF's nose! Mom: 42-years-old with severe job stress. She had known she had another baby there for approximately 9 years. She'd experienced several miscarriages, failed IVF; she had high FSH, low AMH, and an absence of cervical mucus. This woman is a Sensitive and I was one of the only therapists to acknowledge it and to support it. (She did have a male healer friend who did so as well.) It was actually crucial to her success because she had a great deal of information and trusting and validating it enhanced its potency.

Together we did about 2 dozen sessions: fertility, birth, and then beyond over about a 2-year timeframe. A month or so into our work my client had a dream that she would have a baby girl and the baby would be born on a particular football Sunday. I totally believed that and I told her so. As we worked together she was able to better trust her intuition and her Sensitive abilities. We cleared various blocks which enabled her to better engage the 3 keys: meditate, listen, and trust. That's exactly what she did and her baby girl was born on the very Sunday she had dreamed of nearly a year before.

On the waiting list for IVF, before her turn came my client was naturally pregnant. She was elated and other things came together in her life as well. She was having a horrendous time at her job and she was able to get a lengthy paid leave and then, eventually, not go back. She called my office during her pregnancy to say she had a placenta previa and we set up a Skype session to address it. Through the power of precision hypnosis my client and I took care of it and she was able to have the natural, vaginal birth she desired. Her healthy baby girl was received into the world by joyful parents (though they did miss a football game) on a blustery November day. A new sparkly orb is aligning right now with my client and her little family.

Case K

I worked with a 40-year-old client from overseas for 12 sessions by phone; I did see her in person once when she was in the Denver area. This client had endured 5 failed IVFs, a miscarriage, and the termination of a Downs baby at 12 weeks. By the time she met with me this woman had several frozen embryos and a plan to transfer 3. The doctor was resistant to transferring 3 but my client insisted as each of her other IVFs had failed when only 1 or 2 embryos were transferred. Her main issue was stress and fear—fear, in particular, of having to do another amniocentesis (and getting further bad news).

I helped my client to clear subconscious traumas, and any blocks that may have arisen. She was originally from the United States so was a great distance from family and childhood friends, also more traditional customs and her familiar culture. She'd endured some severe criticism from a family member and friend or two regarding her choice to terminate the Downs pregnancy. Truly that was hers and her husband's choice to make whether or not anyone agrees with it. I held the space, provided support, and guided her through her process at her own pace.

After a few sessions my client had her embryo transfer. She held fast with the doctor and received 3 healthy embryos. She really only wanted one baby at a time so we put that into her sessions. My client became pregnant with one healthy baby girl. I worked with her to pass the critical time and her husband was very supportive. Once she knew she had a healthy baby girl she floated through her pregnancy quite comfortably; I did a bit to help with NVP (nausea and vomiting during pregnancy) early on and then some healing work to support rapid recovery from an elective c-section.

Case L

When I met this 44-year-old client she was on her 3rd and last transfer. She'd had a lifelong struggle with depression, and she'd had an abortion years earlier that was unresolved. This woman had a high stress job as a project manager; she was athletic and said she got along much better with men than with women. She had some childhood issues, a main one being that her mother had basically just "quit" being a mother right around the time my client entered puberty. This was significant.

This client and I focused quite a bit on the Divine Feminine; on embracing the feminine; on feminine attributes and philosophy, rites and rituals. This type of work powerfully impacts the subconscious mind which, as you'll recall, responds to metaphor, story, and emotion. There was a balance occurring here but it was different than some of the more standard interpretation. She was balancing her psyche: male/female, yin/yang, anima/animus. This client especially needed to cultivate receptivity; to nurture herself so that she could deeply nurture another.

All in all I spent about 15 sessions with this client. She really embraced and honored her process—it was not always easy but she did it. Virtually existing in a man's world, doing things as men do, she, as do other women in similar situations, had buried her authentic self, her individual Divine self—also the Divine Mother. Most of my clients are Type-A personalities as I have mentioned, and I typically address such traits with them if only for the sheer purpose of amalgamation of method. Self-esteem tends to take a hit during infertility; for clients navigating the staggering minuet of tiptoeing, sidestepping, schmoozing, and—as necessary—head-butting alpha males, self-esteem and energy levels often plummet.

I worked with my client to integrate the tools and skills she had acquired along her life path, though in some cases to put a different spin on them. She was amazed at how interactions with some of what she thought of as female-phobic co-workers became more respectful, sometimes even friendlier. *The energy shifted* was what she told me. And she was right—there is an energy shift that occurs when we do this type of work; for conception purposes that shift is exactly the energy alignment the spirit babies have been referencing.

Huge changes occurred for this client—in her career, and in her relationship. She and her husband became parents to a darling little daughter, and she was beyond thrilled that she had done the feminine/mother work so that she could share it with—and eventually teach it to—her own little girl.

Chapter 89

LIFE'S GREATEST ACCOMPLISHMENT

"I said to my soul, be still, and wait without hope.
For hope would be hope for the wrong thing; and wait without love, for
love would be love of the wrong thing; there is yet faith. But the faith, and
the hope, and the love are all in the waiting.
And so the darkness shall be the light, and the stillness, the dancing."

—*T. S. Eliot*

I can honestly say that my most important
accomplishment is my children. I am a go-getter, Type-A
personality; I am creative, driven, and self-motivated. I could
certainly be called an over-achiever: I have acquired various
degrees and certifications throughout my life; I have achieved
certain status and position. I continue to do so because I have
a great love of learning and a great love of living. I have at the
same time managed to balance my overall mind, body, spirit so
as not to be overextending myself or creating burnout induced
illness or issue.

This is precisely why it is so important to me to help
others. I understand achievement and drive, and all that goes
with it, and I also understand that none of it means a thing if
your true desire is to have a baby and you don't have one.
There are women who choose not to have children, who

sincerely do not want to have them. I admire their acknowledgement and acceptance of their own personal truth, their own reality. And because I know your truth I want to share it. I have always known this to be something akin to a Universal law—that for those of us who have the burning desire to have children there is no substitute.

I saw this clearly a few years ago when I attended a class at Regis University called *Women Transforming the World*. One of the books we were assigned to read is called *In Sweet Company* (Wolff, 2004). This brilliant book leads us into the hearts, minds, and lives of several influential and spiritual women; women who are committed to making a difference in this world. As I read each of the inspirational stories I was struck by how often when asked what they considered their greatest accomplishment, the answers from the women with children reflected what I knew to be true for me: their children.

Following are a few quotes from this most impressive writing:

Grandmother Twylah Hurd Nitsch (p. 32) said: "If you were to ask me about my greatest experience, I would say being married and raising my five children."

Miriam Polster (p. 48) is quoted as saying: ". . . I think raising two decent, ethical human beings is one of my greatest accomplishments."

Olympia Dukakis was also interviewed (p. 101). Her response was: "That I had children, raised them, and somehow we held it together in the midst of some horrendous things that happened."

And Rabbi Laura Gellar (p. 200) said: "I'm not sure I can answer that. I love being a mother."

I do not believe that every woman on the planet is supposed to have a baby or that there is anything wrong with anyone who doesn't. I simply know that for those who do have the desire, it is strong. It is emotionally driven and it is genetically driven—after all, our strongest human instinct is to procreate. This matters so much to me; this is my life's work. I have facilitated the connection between thousands of babies and mothers, and I will continue to do so.

A mother's love is often conveyed through analogies of bears or lions. The child is the absolute center of the Universe—mother's life is but to be given in exchange for the life of her baby. Ferocious—as with a bear or lion—the fight to the death against any and all enemies is express and implied. We would die for our babies—and we would do so gladly. It is this deep and indisputable instinct that enables us to lay down our lives for them; and it is what drives us to the brink just to have one in the first place.

Joseph Campbell, the world renowned mythologist, studied—for more than half a century—myths, symbols, archetypes, stories, and cultures from around the globe and spanning thousands of years. Joseph Campbell is not known for mincing words or concerning himself with how others might react to his discoveries. He has one of the world's most brilliant minds and has used it to unravel some of the earth's most knotted yarns, and to draw indisputable parallels from one culture, one time period, to the next. In a lecture series he gave entitled *The Power of Myth* Campbell gives us profound insight into the very subject we have been addressing here, and into the human psyche:

"As soon as you beget or give birth to a child, you're the dead one. The child is the new life and you are simply the protector of that new life."

I hope that this book has been helpful to you—and to all the spirit babies who are my inspiration. I am grateful to have been able to share this information with you, to encourage you, and hopefully to even enlighten you. Your baby(s) is coming to you in just the right time, and in just the right way . . . remember the 3 keys: meditate, listen, trust.

As a team, we Earth angels, Lightworkers, Indigos, Crystals, Rainbows and whatever generations that God/Goddess has in store for us after that, are all here working together. We're all here for peace. And we can do it!

—*Doreen Virtue*

AFTERWORD

As this book was in its editing phase miracles continued to unfold in my practice. A client who had never been pregnant—had experienced seven failed IVFs (some donor, some not) on top of countless other unsuccessful attempts to conceive—became pregnant. Her fertility journey had started ten years ago. This client adopted a little boy from overseas some five or so years ago, and her son has been telling her from the time he could speak that he has a little sister. When she mentioned this to me early on in our sessions I told her that I take it as a good sign—eventually I out and out told her that my "money's on *Westin."

Westin used to talk to his sister all the time but hadn't in over a year. He is at that age where kids naturally tend to stop that kind of interaction. About three days before her embryo transfer, my client's son began talking to his sister again. I knew that baby was coming and that piece of information clinched it for me. My client really wanted to believe it but with that brutal ten-year journey under her belt she wasn't totally there.

She knows about Dylan's gifts so between sessions I mentioned my client's first name only to Dylan. He instantly told me her hair and eye color, described her physical essence, and said that she is bringing in a girl—and a precocious one at that. Well, now Dylan and Westin—obviously still very connected to that world—were in agreement. I told my client and she was quite pleased to hear what Dylan had said. As I opened my daytimer to record the date of her pregnancy test I discovered it to be the day of Dylan's eighteenth birthday. I shared that with my client as just one more sign.

Two days later I received a joyful voicemail from Westin and his little sister's mom. She is pregnant! She thanked me and said some very kind and appreciative words to Dylan—I had him listen to the voicemail so he could hear them for himself. This woman had been ready to use a surrogate but after beginning her hypnotherapy sessions with me she went in and her doctors told her something had changed; they recommended she give it another try herself. My client told me she only did one thing different: hypnosis.

During the first (sometimes the second) session I tell my new clients: we are going to have a conversation a little ways down the road and we are going to remember the one we are having now. You're going to bring your baby to my office or let me see him/her by Skype. And we're going to talk about how far off all this seemed to you when we first met. This conversation will happen and you're going to have to laugh when it does.

This is my favorite part of the work I do and I look forward to it immensely. And I do have these conversations— over and over I have the privilege of witnessing the process come full circle, of seeing the sheer delight in my clients' eyes as they show me their sweet, adorable babies; as they stand or sit before me, energy glowing, proudly exhibiting their hard earned—but well worth it all—badge of honor: **MOTHER.**

*Westin's name has been changed as his first name is unique and too easily identifiable to include here.

TESTIMONIALS

Some of these testimonials are also available on my web site (SpiritBabyWhisperer.com). I include just a few here because I believe they are invaluable to those on this fertility journey . . .

I was 43-years-old and struggling with secondary infertility. I already had a beautiful 2-year-old daughter but I just couldn't conceive again. The doctors were talking about "advanced maternal age" and suggesting I go with donor eggs. But, I just couldn't. I knew there was a baby there (just like it says in Lynsi's book!) and I needed to explore that possibility. People are often unkind to women with secondary infertility. They figure we should be happy we have one child and just leave it alone. But I just can't convey how painful it is to have only one baby who may never have any siblings; to be unable to choose when your family is complete.

I tried everything: acupuncture, herbs, chiropractic, yoga, change in diet, etc. But nothing was working and I kept beating myself up. My acupuncturist gave me a copy of It's Conceivable!, and I resonated with it right away. I just knew I had to get in touch with Lynsi and I called her office right away. I was thrilled to learn that she took clients by telephone and Skype as well as in person. I was able to get started within about a week and Lynsi and I worked through 3 ovulation cycles. I continued my acupuncture, herbs, yoga, and diet and I was pleased that Lynsi said the hypnosis would complement the other work I was doing, including medical treatment if I chose to have it. Lynsi said she and the other practitioners were my support team and I did feel very supported and grateful. By the 11th session I was naturally pregnant! I continued with my support team on what Lynsi calls an "as needed" basis, and in March 2009 gave birth to a beautiful baby girl, Emily Anne! The hypnosis helped make the birth a comfortable and joyful process as well. I had a natural birth and was up and around quickly. Lynsi, I want to thank you from the bottom of my heart. I don't believe this could have happened without you.

—Aubrey
Austin, TX

I was a bit of a hysterical mess when I went in to see Lynsi Eastburn. I was 42-years-old, and the doctors had given me less than 1% chance of conception and practically ordered me to do donor eggs. I was stunned. This was not what I'd expected to hear that day in the doctor's office. I did NOT wish to do donor eggs and I told Lynsi so. She honored my wishes and told me we would start from where I was. We worked on getting me into a state of mind/body/spirit balance where, she explained, I could make any decisions I needed to make regarding my fertility. I honestly felt like I was about to crack from everything I'd been through with the doctors, but Lynsi handled my fragile emotions gently and considerately. I believe it was the sense of safety I experienced in her office that helped me keep it together.

After about 3 sessions I realized that I had made a decision— that I wanted to do donor eggs! It just came up from the depths of my subconscious which was now a much calmer and friendlier place to be. I was in balance: mind/body/spirit. I was amazed to find out that not only did I want to do donor eggs but that I was excited about the process! My husband and I picked a donor, and within a few months we were on our way! We ended up with 2 embryos and transferred both of them. We were nervous that there were only two but Lynsi reminded us that everything is as it should be and sure enough, we ended up with twins! At the age of 43 I gave birth to a healthy baby girl and boy via c-section. And thanks to the hypnosis we continued throughout the pregnancy my c-section was a breeze and my recovery rapid.

I'd just like to say that no matter what kind of turmoil you are in around your fertility, there is hope and there is help! Lynsi really gets it and she can help you bring your baby(s) into this world "in just the right time and in just the right way" as she always says. Good luck!

—Susan
Aurora, CO

I have been on the infertility journey for 6 years. After five IVF cycles I was left with one normal 3-day embryo ready for transfer. I knew this was our final IVF cycle, which only added to our anxiety. I am an engineer, an analytical type, with a Type-A personality. I knew that I had selected the best doctors and had a normal embryo. Now I needed to make sure I was not interfering by over thinking everything.

I had heard of doing hypnosis during infertility treatments and after some research learned of Lynsi Eastburn. After a call to her office, I arranged four "meetings"—one in person in Colorado, and three via telephone (because I lived out of state). For the telephone "meetings" Lynsi provided hypnosis recordings that I listened to every evening. Our meetings were excellent and I really felt that she provided customized hypnosis that really spoke to me, both my situation and my concerns.

One of the things that I think made the biggest difference in preparing myself mentally for the frozen embryo transfer was doing hypnosis with Lynsi. I was a wreck after our "zero normals" result in November. I was sobbing and breaking down at anything. I was in terrible shape. Considering where I was mentally, I think my change in attitude made all the difference. Some women can do it themselves, but I needed outside intervention and Lynsi provided it. The hypnosis really helped me put my feet on the ground. I felt at peace with the outcome and I NEVER felt that before. After the transfer I really took it easy, and continued listening to the hypnosis recordings Lynsi did for me.

After years of heartbreak and disappointment, my husband and I are in a place filled with hope and joy. I am now 23 weeks pregnant and truly believe this was only possible with the help of Lynsi.

—Jennifer
Detroit, Michigan

*Update: a beautiful Christmas card picture update of Jennifer, her husband, and their little daughter arrived at my office just last month.

By the time I arrived in Lynsi's office, I was 33 years old and I had been trying to have a baby for 3 ½ years. In those 3 ½ years, I had one miscarriage from a spontaneous pregnancy and a miscarriage from an IVF. I had tried everything under the sun to conceive a child including acupuncture, diet changes, putting my legs up the wall after sex, IUIs, IVFs, surgeries for endometriosis, and none of it worked. Furthermore, no one could give me a really good reason why I couldn't get pregnant. I was despondent, depressed, but desperate to have the child my husband and I had wanted for so long. I figured I had absolutely nothing to lose by trying HypnoFertility®—it felt like a last resort, but the worst that could happen was it wouldn't work. I walked into Lynsi's office and told her "I am doing a frozen embryo transfer in a month and I do not want you to tell me to wait!" Lynsi didn't even blink an eye at my abrupt statement, she just said "OK—let's work with that." I think it was the first time in 3 ½ years that doctors, acupuncturists and therapists hadn't dictated a time frame to me—I already liked that.

I went once a week to Lynsi prior to embryo transfer and once a week through the transfer process. I realized the pervasive message I received was that my body was broken and I couldn't get pregnant. And frankly, my subconscious believed it as well. Lynsi and I worked through changing that belief and throughout the process my mantra was "Things are happening exactly the way they should." This helped relieve the anxiety of going through assisted reproductive technologies. And sure enough, two weeks later, the doctor called with the news that I was pregnant! I was terrified of miscarriage and I saw Lynsi throughout my whole pregnancy to relieve the miscarriage anxiety. On August 4, 2010, I gave birth to a beautiful baby girl, Francesca Marie.

But our story doesn't end there. The benefits of my work with Lynsi continued on when I discovered I was pregnant naturally with baby #2 just 6 months after Francesca was born! Something mentally had shifted in me after doing HypnoFertility®, and I never doubted that I could get pregnant with #2. Thanks to Lynsi's work with me, I feel hopeful and fearless in this pregnancy. And I sit here now due with a baby boy in November 2011 and feel eternally grateful for the work Lynsi and I did together. She helped changed my thought patterns, the view of my body, and gave me the confidence to be an advocate in my fertility. Although the initial goal of hypnosis was to get pregnant, I found that I gained much more in terms of managing my anxiety, having new hope, and finding purpose again in my life after struggling with my fertility so long. There will never be enough good things to say about the benefits of working with Lynsi!

—Tricia
Denver, CO

Trying to conceive was one of the hardest times of my life. Once my husband and I were ready to start a family in our early 30s, we tried for 6 months without success. I then went in for an evaluation to get some reassurance that everything was alright, but instead I got the most devastating news of my life. I was told I would be unable to get pregnant

204

naturally due to a low ovarian reserve and limited time of fertility left. It was recommended to start fertility treatments right away.

At first I was hopeful that fertility treatments would help me to get pregnant, but after 3 failed intrauterine inseminations depression and feeling that I would never get pregnant set in. The next step was to have IVF. Before the IVF, I knew that I needed to put myself in a better place or all of the stress that I was feeling would not be beneficial.

I saw Lynsi for only one visit before my first IVF round, and even with only one visit I could already feel a sense of hope beginning to come back. However, all of this was again dashed after my IVF round was cancelled due to a poor response. After this happened I again went into a feeling of hopelessness, but knew how important it was to continue to see Lynsi to help decrease my stress.

Each session with Lynsi was a wonderful experience. I always left feeling a sense of peace and hope. I also began to listen to her recordings at home, which helped to reinforce her teachings. I was preparing to start my 2nd round of IVF when I got a great surprise, I was pregnant! After being told I would never get pregnant naturally I couldn't believe that I was pregnant without any fertility treatments and would be able to start the family I had longed for.

Looking back, I know that I could have not done this without Lynsi's help. I noticed a change in myself over the short 3 months that I was seeing her, and really feel that this led to a natural pregnancy. Thank you Lynsi for all of your help, I will always be grateful.

—Wendy
Castle Rock, CO

My wife and I had been through so much when we came to Lynsi Eastburn. She helped us heal the past and believe we could have a healthy baby. Now we have our healthy 11-month-old boy and we could not have had such an experience without you. You helped bring the ease back to our relationship as well. Can't thank you enough.

—Aaron
Portland, OR

After several pregnancy losses, turning 40, and 2 reproductive endocrinologists—the list goes on . . . I finally let go and decided to see

Lynsi Easturn. I am a Hypnotherapist but knew I needed to go to the best one I could find. I was so impressed with Lynsi that I decided to fly to Denver to see her privately, and also take her HypnoFertility® training. I had two private sessions before the weekend training, then came home and one week later found out I was pregnant! It took me 5 years to get here but just one life changing weekend with Lynsi. I will forever remember her care and support. There is a reason why people need to specialize and so I have modeled her approach and now have the honor of helping other women and men who struggle with fertility issues. My son is the most calm and easy going boy you could ever meet. This is a typical hypnobaby. My husband and I are grateful to Lynsi forever.

We love you, Lynsi, and our boy is the greatest match for us, thank you!!!

—*Clare Katner, LMT, Hypnotherapist*
Portland, OR

Update: A few months ago I received a thrilling voicemail from a very excited Clare. She and Aaron (above) were 12 weeks naturally pregnant. This was supposed to be impossible and the couple had accepted that, and were truly happy with their baby son. Surprise! Congratulations, Clare & Aaron!

Hi Lynsi,

I've been meaning to contact you and let you know that our baby Adrian is here and it's been 6 months now and I realized I still hadn't done that! I'm so sorry. I wanted to thank you for the hypnosis and your help in our journey to bring him here. We made a website for him so you can see pictures of him. So he's here and healthy as can be and that's all that matters. We're absolutely crazy about him. Thanks again for your help and support!!

—*Valerie*
Denver, CO

When I first met Lynsi my husband and I had been struggling for 3 years with infertility. After 3 failed IVFs, I came to a realization: while doctors played an important role in providing the technical means to get pregnant, they were not getting me any closer to my dream, nor were they giving me hope that another cycle would work.

That's when I discovered the healing power of complementary therapists like Lynsi. These special individuals not only were truly effective at bringing me closer to my dream (for example, by significantly lowering my FSH and reversing my biological clock in a way that doctors could not—yes, it CAN be done!) but also tended to my heart and mind. While doctors addressed my medical requirements, these people truly listened to me, looked me straight in the eye and said, "Yes you can have a baby." They gave me hope.

Lynsi is just such a special person. She helped me to feel confident during an otherwise uncertain time. She helped me to counter negative programming and to conceive that not only was having a baby possible, it was inevitable. If you believe that reducing your anxiety can improve your likelihood of success, Lynsi can help you. Beyond that if you believe that what you conceive of internally can be manifested physically, or that connecting with your child can help bring your child to you, Lynsi can help you.

I once heard Lynsi say that anyone who wants a baby should have one. I believe Lynsi has a gift that goes beyond medical science—an ability to bring children together with the parents who desire them. And whenever I hold my precious son in my arms I feel grateful for this gift and for Lynsi's help along my way.

—L.R., 41
San Francisco Bay Area

Hey Lynsi, just wanted to formally announce: it's a boy!!! And to say thanks for your help, I was so worried when the contractions started at only 27 weeks but the work we did together kept the baby in till 38 weeks and that was even better than what the doctors were hoping for. I know you work mostly with fertility but you were a Godsend to us in keeping our baby from being born too early. Now he has the best start to life, and I highly recommend your services. Thanks again, Lynsi!

—Joanne
Lakewood, CO

ABOUT THE AUTHOR

Lynsi Eastburn is a registered psychotherapist, NGH Board Certified Hypnotherapist and Certified Instructor. She is co-owner and instructor—along with her husband, Drake—of the Eastburn Institute of Hypnosis and Eastburn Hypnotherapy Center in Colorado, a faculty member of several hypnosis organizations, and also runs a full time private practice. Lynsi has been featured nationally on *The Balancing Act* on *Lifetime Television Network*, *ABC* and *CBS News*, on national and international radio programs, and in print media including *The Denver Post, The Rocky Mountain News, Cosmopolitan Pregnancy Magazine,* and *Conceive Magazine.*

Lynsi is the creator of HypnoFertility®—a program based on clinical experience gleaned from thousands of hours in her Colorado private practice—she has taught her methods internationally. She is the recipient of awards—including the *Education and Literature Award* and the National Guild of Hypnotists' prestigious *Hypnosis Research Award (2005)*—for her groundbreaking work in the fertility hypnosis field.

Lynsi is the author of *It's Conceivable!*, an unprecedented book chronicling various success stories of her private clients. Her new book *The 3 Keys to Conception* was released in February 2013, and a new edition of *It's Conceivable!* is also in the works. Lynsi is president of the Denver NGH chapter.

Originally from Toronto, Canada, Lynsi currently lives in Colorado with her husband, Drake, son, Dylan, and two dogs, Boo Radley and Scout. Her older son, Kelly, is living in Toronto.

Lynsi & Drake are thrilled to be grandparents to a little boy expected in April 2013. Congratulations to Coady & Kylie!

Take Action!

The Eastburn motto is Change Your Mind, Change Your Life. *The Eastburn hypnotism training is called the* Transformational Hypnotherapy Certification *program. There is a reason for this. Drake & Lynsi Eastburn have dedicated their lives to the mastery of the art and science of hypnotism and its powerful applications in the mind/body/spirit healing arena. With more than 50 years combined experience they are the global go-to source for those desiring quality, cutting edge hypnotherapy sessions, workshops, and certification training. Both Drake & Lynsi Eastburn have logged literally tens of thousands of clinic and teaching hours over the course of their careers; they are committed to the success of their clients and students and for that reason—as well as their own self-growth—they are also lifelong learners.*

You and your children's futures are determined by the choices you make today, by what you decide to do with the knowledge you gleaned from this reading. What does your gut tell you? Do something? Don't do something? Keep the keys in mind whatever the case: meditate, listen, trust. The choice for healing, for mind/body/spirit balance, for creating what you want in your life, is yours. And only yours.

Available at Eastburn Hypnotherapy Center:

By Lynsi Eastburn:

- *It's Conceivable! Hypnosis for Fertility*
- *The 3 Keys to Conception: Pregnancy Against All Odds*
- *Natural Conception and IVF Assistant CD sets*

Soon to be Announced . . . Fertility Retreats
in Tulum, Mexico
with Lynsi Eastburn and Shelley Torgrove
More information will appear on the web sites as it becomes
available. *November 2013.*

By Drake Eastburn:

- The Power of the Past: *Transformational Replay: State-of-the-art Hypnotic Regression Therapy*
- Power Patter: *A Script Book for Hypnotists*
- No Time to Waist: Powerful Weight Loss Secrets You Need to Know *(Book + 6 CD Complete Weight Loss Program)*
- What is Hypnosis? (Really): What Every Person Should Know About Hypnosis
- The Power of Suggestion
- The Therapeutic Hypnotist *(soon to be released)*

And with Drake and/or Lynsi:

- *In office, telephone, and Skype hypnotherapy/HypnoFertility® sessions*
- *On site and distance certification training and advanced classes*
- *Weight, stress reduction, self-hypnosis, smoking cessation seminars*
- *Advanced training DVDs including:*
  - **Working with the Esdaile State:** *Resolving Body-Focused Repetitive Behaviors (Impulse Control Disorders) Through the Esdaile State. [10 CEUs]*
  - **Hypnotic Regression:** Power of the Past: *learn to address and release a variety of issues, from phobias and weight control to smoking cessation, performance enhancement, and much more. [32 CEUs]*
  - **Instant and Rapid Inductions and Hypnotic Depth Testing:** *How to efficiently and effectively get hypnotic analgesia and anesthesia. [8 CEUs]*
  - **Working with Sleep Issues** *[3 CEUs]*

Powerful Hypnosis CDs
Achieve Incredible Results Effortlessly!

Titles Include:

- *Stress Reduction CD*
- *Weight Mastery CD*
- *Nighttime Weight Loss CD*
- *Metabolism I & II*
- *Appetite Recognition CD*
- *Youth Weight Mastery (Daytime/Nighttime)*
- *HypnoFertility® General Healing CD*
- *Prosperity (Daytime/Nighttime)*
- *Lift Your Spirits (Daytime/Nighttime)*
- *Non-Smoker for Life CD*
- *Relax, Rejuvenate, Renew CD*
- *Healing Rain Song CD*
- *Ferrel Rest CD*
- *Cat Purr for Healing CD*
- *Nighttime Healing CD*

**Eastburn Institute of Hypnosis
& Eastburn Hypnotherapy Center
7905 N. Zenobia St.
Westminster, CO 80030**

(303) 424-2331

www.hypnofertility.com

www.SpiritBabyWhisperer.com

www.hypnodenver.com

REFERENCES

Benson, H. (1975). *The relaxation response: The classic mind/body approach that has helped millions conquer the harmful effects of stress.* New York, NY: Harper Collins.

Bolte Taylor, J. (2006). *My stroke of insight: A brain scientist's personal journey.* New York, NY: Viking Penguin.

Calhoun, M. (2002). *Are you really too sensitive?* Citrus Heights, CA: Intuitive Development Publishing.

Causton, R. (1995). *The Buddha in daily life: An introduction to the Buddhism of Nichiren Daishonin.* London, UK: Random House.

de Becker, G. (1997). *The gift of fear: And other survival signals that protect us from violence.* New York, NY: Dell Publishing.

Eastburn, D., E. (2010). *What is hypnosis?: Really.* Denver, CO: D. James Publishing.

Eastburn, L., J. (2006). *It's conceivable!: Hypnosis for fertility.* Victoria, BC: Trafford Publishing.

Fields, R., Weyler, R., Ingrasci, R., & Taylor, P. (1984). *Chop wood carry water: A guide to finding spiritual fulfillment in daily life.* Los Angeles, CA: Jeremy P. Tarcher, Inc.

Hanh, T. N. (2001). *Anger: Wisdom for cooling the flames.* New York, NY: Penguin Group (USA), Inc.

Hanson, R. (2009). *Buddha's brain: The practical neuroscience of happiness, love, and wisdom.* Oakland, CA: New Harbinger Publications, Inc.

REFERENCES

Herman, J. (1997). *Trauma and recovery: The aftermath of violence— from domestic abuse to political terror.* New York, NY: Basic Books.

Horton, C. (2006). *Revenge of the wounded child.* Golden, CO: Higher Self Workshops.

Johnson, A. (2012). Let go of control: How to use the art of surrender. Retrieved from: http://www.tinybuddha.com

Lipton, B. (2005). *The biology of belief: unleashing the power of consciousness, matter & miracles.* New York, NY: Hay House.

Losey Blackburn, M. (2007). *The children of now.* Franklin Lakes, NJ: New Page Books.

Makichen, W. (2005). *Spirit babies: How to communicate with the child you're meant to have.* New York, NY: Bantam Dell.

Miller, A. (1997). *The drama of the gifted child: The search for the true self.* New York, NY: Basic Books.

Surrender. 2012. In *Merriam-Webster.com.* Retrieved November 12, 2012, from http://www.merriam-webster.com/dictionary/surrender

Virtue, D. (2010). Indigo, crystal and rainbow children. Retrieved from: http://www.angeltherapy.com/article1.php

REFERENCES

Weiss, B. L. (1988). *Many lives, many masters.* New York, NY: Simon & Schuster.

Weiss, B. L. (2000). *Messages from the masters: Tapping into the power of love.* New York, NY: Warner Books, Inc.

Woodman, M. (1985). *The pregnant virgin: A process of psychological transformation.* Toronto, ON: Inner City Books.

Wolff, M. (2004). *In sweet company: Conversations with extraordinary women about living a spiritual life.* San Francisco, CA: Jossey-Bass.